T0227019

Advances in the Management of Benign Esophageal Diseases

Guest Editor

BLAIR A. JOBE, MD

THORACIC SURGERY CLINICS

www.thoracic.theclinics.com

Consulting Editor
MARK K. FERGUSON, MD

November 2011 • Volume 21 • Number 4

SAUNDERS an imprint of ELSEVIER, Inc.

W.B. SAUNDERS COMPANY
A Division of Elsevier Inc.

1600 John F. Kennedy Boulevard • Suite 1800 • Philadelphia, Pennsylvania 19103-2899

http://www.theclinics.com

THORACIC SURGERY CLINICS Volume 21, Number 4
November 2011 ISSN 1547-4127, ISBN-13: 978-1-4557-1159-8

Editor: Barbara Cohen-Kligerman

Thoracic Surgery Clinics (ISSN 1547-4127) is published quarterly by Elsevier Inc., 360 Park Avenue South, New York, NY 10010-1710. Months of publication are February, May, August, and November. Business and editorial offices: 1600 John F. Kennedy Boulevard, Suite 1800, Philadelphia, PA 19103-2899. Periodicals postage paid at New York, NY, and additional mailing offices. Subscription prices are $295.00 per year (US individuals), $385.00 per year (US institutions), $141.00 per year (US Students), $367.00 per year (Canadian individuals), $487.00 per year (Canadian institutions), $192.00 per year (Canadian and foreign students), $391.00 per year (foreign individuals), and $487.00 per year (foreign institutions). Foreign air speed delivery is included in all Clinics' subscription prices. All prices are subject to change without notice. **POSTMASTER:** Send address changes to Thoracic Surgery Clinics, Elsevier Health Sciences Division, Subscription Customer Service, 3251 Riverport Lane, Maryland Heights, MO 63043. **Customer Service (orders, claims, online, change of address): Telephone: 1-800-654-2452 (U.S. and Canada); 314-447-8871 (outside U.S. and Canada). Fax: 314-447-8029. Email: journalscustomerservice-usa@elsevier.com (for print support); journalsonlinesupport-usa@elsevier.com (for online support).**

Reprints. For copies of 100 or more, of articles in this publication, please contact Commercial Rights Department, Elsevier Inc., 360 Park Avenue South, New York, NY 10010-1710. Tel: (212) 633-3812; Fax: (212) 462-1935; E-mail: reprints@elsevier.com.

Thoracic Surgery Clinics is covered in *MEDLINE/PubMed (Index Medicus)* and *EMBASE/Excerpta Medica.*

Printed and bound by CPI Group (UK) Ltd, Croydon, CR0 4YY

Transferred to Digital Print 2011

Contributors

CONSULTING EDITOR

MARK K. FERGUSON, MD
Professor of Surgery, Section of Cardiac and
Thoracic Surgery, The University of Chicago
Medical Center, Chicago, Illinois

GUEST EDITOR

BLAIR A. JOBE, MD, FACS
Professor of Surgery, Division of Thoracic and
Foregut Surgery, Department of
Cardiothoracic Surgery, University of
Pittsburgh Medical Center, Pittsburgh,
Pennsylvania

AUTHORS

**DAVID ARMSTRONG, MA, MB BChir,
FRCP(UK), AGAF, FRCPC**
Associate Professor, Division of
Gastroenterology, McMaster University,
Hamilton, Ontario, Canada

PHILIP W. CARROTT Jr, MD, FACS
Ryan Hill Thoraco-esophageal Fellow,
Department of Surgery, Virginia Mason
Medical Center, Seattle, Washington

TOSHITAKA HOPPO, MD, PhD
Research Assistant Professor, Division
of Thoracic and Foregut Surgery,
Department of Cardiothoracic Surgery,
University of Pittsburgh Medical Center,
Pittsburgh, Pennsylvania

TOSHIHISA HOSOYA, MD
Digestive Disease Center, Showa University
Northern Yokohama Hospital, Tsuzuki-ku,
Yokohama, Japan

JOHN G. HUNTER, MD
Mackenzie Professor and Chairman,
Department of Surgery, Oregon Health &
Sciences University, Portland, Oregon

HARUO IKEDA, MD
Digestive Disease Center, Showa University
Northern Yokohama Hospital, Tsuzuki-ku,
Yokohama, Japan

HARUHIRO INOUE, MD, PhD, FASGE
Digestive Disease Center, Showa University
Northern Yokohama Hospital, Tsuzuki-ku,
Yokohama, Japan

BLAIR A. JOBE, MD, FACS
Professor of Surgery, Division of Thoracic
and Foregut Surgery, Department of
Cardiothoracic Surgery, University of
Pittsburgh Medical Center, Pittsburgh,
Pennsylvania

SHIN-EI KUDO, MD, PhD
Digestive Disease Center, Showa University
Northern Yokohama Hospital, Tsuzuki-ku,
Yokohama, Japan

YONG S. KWON, MD
Department of Surgery, Center for
Videoendoscopic Surgery, University of
Washington, Seattle, Washington

DONALD E. LOW, MD, FACS, FRCS(C)
Head, Thoracic Oncology and Thoracic
Surgery, Department of Surgery, Virginia
Mason Medical Center; Clinical Assistant
Professor of Surgery, University of Washington
School of Medicine, Seattle, Washington

ALBERT L. MERATI, MD
Professor, Department of Otolaryngology,
University of Washington, Seattle,
Washington

HITOMI MINAMI, MD
Digestive Disease Center, Showa University
Northern Yokohama Hospital, Tsuzuki-ku,
Yokohama, Japan

BRANT K. OELSCHLAGER, MD
Director and Byers Endowed Professor of
Esophageal Research, Department of Surgery,
Center for Videoendoscopic Surgery,
University of Washington, Seattle,
Washington

MANABU ONIMARU, MD, PhD
Digestive Disease Center, Showa University
Northern Yokohama Hospital, Tsuzuki-ku,
Yokohama, Japan

JOHN E. PANDOLFINO, MD
Department of Medicine, Feinberg School
of Medicine, Northwestern University,
Chicago, Illinois

SHAH D. RACHIT, MD
Clinical Instructor, Division of Thoracic and
Foregut Surgery, Department of
Cardiothoracic Surgery, University of
Pittsburgh Medical Center, Pittsburgh,
Pennsylvania

KEVIN M. REAVIS, MD, FACS
Assistant Professor of Clinical Surgery, Division
of Gastrointestinal Surgery, Department of
Surgery, Irvine Medical Center, University of
California, Orange; Veterans Affairs Healthcare
System Long Beach, Long Beach, California

SABINE ROMAN, MD, PhD
Digestive Physiology, Edouard Herriot
Hospital, Hospices Civils de Lyon, Université
Claude Bernard Lyon I, Lyon, France

DANIEL SIFRIM, MD, PhD
Professor of GI Physiology, Director of Upper
GI Physiology Unit, Barts and The London
School of Medicine and Dentistry, Wingate
Institute of Neurogastroenterology, London,
United Kingdom

ALEX STRAUMANN, MD
Chairman, Swiss EoE-Research Group, Olten;
Professor, Department of Gastroenterology,
University Hospital Basel, Basel, Switzerland

KRIS MA TIANLE, MD, PhD
Digestive Disease Center, Showa University
Northern Yokohama Hospital, Tsuzuki-ku,
Yokohama, Japan

BRANDON H. TIEU, MD
Assistant Professor of Surgery, Division of
Cardiothoracic Surgery, Oregon Health &
Sciences University, Portland, Oregon

THOMAS J. WATSON, MD, FACS
Associate Professor of Surgery, Chief of
Thoracic Surgery, University of Rochester
School of Medicine and Dentistry,
Rochester, New York

AKIRA YOSHIDA, MD, PhD
Digestive Disease Center, Showa University
Northern Yokohama Hospital, Tsuzuki-ku,
Yokohama, Japan

Contents

procedure does not induce weight loss or treat the comorbid conditions related to obesity. Roux-en-Y gastric bypass is a highly effective treatment of GERD, obesity, and the associated comorbidities. Surgeons who are not comfortable with a bariatric surgical procedure in these patients should either complete appropriate advanced training in bariatric surgery or refer those patients to a qualified surgeon who can offer these options.

The strong association between gastroesophageal reflux disease (GERD) and the development and progression of pulmonary diseases has been suggested, and GERD has been focused on as a potential cause and thus a target for prevention and/or therapy. Because GERD is curable, the proper diagnosis and management of underlying GERD would theoretically improve the outcomes. This article reviews the existing literature and discusses the strategy to manage GERD in patients with end-stage pulmonary diseases before and after lung transplantation.

Cricopharyngeal dysphagia and Zenker 's diverticulum result from cricopharyngeal dysfunction, a failure of the upper esophageal sphincter to relax at the initiation of swallowing. The focus of surgical management involves a cricopharyngeal myotomy that is performed by either an open or an endoscopic approach. The endoscopic approach offers faster operating times, a shorter hospital stay, earlier time to oral intake, and lower complication rates, but a role for open cricopharyngeal myotomy remains.

Peroral endoscopic myotomy (POEM) has been developed as an incisionless, minimally invasive endoscopic treatment intending a permanent cure for esophageal achalasia. The concept of endoscopic myotomy was first reported about 3 decades ago, but the direct incision method through the mucosal layer was not considered to be a safe and reliable approach. A novel method of endoscopic myotomy was developed and established by the authors. In this article, the current techniques, applications, and clinical results of POEM are described.

The management of esophageal high-grade dysplasia (HGD) and intramucosal adenocarcinoma remains controversial. Because lymph node involvement is unlikely in this setting, interest in the treatment strategies for esophageal preservation has grown. Esophageal preservation indicates any endoluminal procedure that is used in an attempt to completely eradicate disease while preserving the anatomic structure of the esophagus. The goal of esophagus-preserving approaches is to provide definitive therapy while avoiding the morbidity of esophagectomy. This article describes the patient selection and the status of currently available esophagus-preserving options, and discusses the strategy for treating HGD and intramusocal adenocarcinoma.

Therapy for acute esophageal perforation in the last decade has benefited from newer technology in endoscopy and imaging. Success with nonoperative therapies such as endoluminal stenting and clipping has improved outcomes and shortened length of stay in selected patients. Iatrogenic injury currently comprises most acute esophageal perforation, and nonoperative therapy may be appropriate in a significant percentage of patients. The decision regarding operative vs non-operative therapy is best done by a dedicated surgical team with experience in all the surgical and endoscopic treatment options. Boerhaave syndrome occurs less often and may be treated with endoscopic therapy, although it more likely requires operative intervention. This article reviews current advances in the diagnosis and management of acute esophageal perforation.

This article highlights current and emerging pharmacological treatments for gastro-esophageal reflux disease (GERD), opportunities for improving medical treatment, the extent to which improvements may be achieved with current therapy, and where new therapies may be required. These issues are discussed in the context of current thinking on the pathogenesis of GERD and its various manifestations and on the pharmacologic basis of current treatments.

Eosinophilic esophagitis is a chronic disease limited to the esophagus and has a persistent or spontaneously fluctuating course. So far it does not seem to limit life expectancy, but it often substantially impairs the quality of life. To date, there has been no association with malignant conditions, but there is concern that the chronic, uncontrolled inflammation will evoke irreversible structural alterations of the esophagus, leading to tissue fibrosis, stricture formation, and impaired function. This esophageal remodeling may result in several disease-inherent and procedure-related complications.

Thoracic Surgery Clinics

READ THE CLINICS ONLINE!

Access your subscription at:
www.theclinics.com

Preface

Advances in the Management of Benign Esophageal Diseases

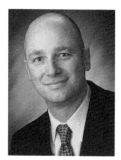

Blair A. Jobe, MD
Guest Editor

In this issue of *Thoracic Surgery Clinics*, an amalgam of the most challenging clinical scenarios in benign esophageal diseases is addressed by experts in the field of esophagology. The recent introduction of novel technologies that have redefined the ways in which we diagnose and treat diseases of the esophagus occupies a prominent place in this issue. For example, an in-depth coverage of high-resolution manometry, a "game changer," along with colored examples of normal and abnormal tracings are provided in a detailed atlas format to serve as a primer and enduring reference. The use of impedance testing in the context of laryngopharyngeal reflux and end-stage lung disease is reviewed and sets the stage for a paradigm shift in our understanding of proximal reflux. Endoscopic imaging in Barrett's esophagus has undergone a revolution and we are ever closer to the "optical biopsy" and the reduction or elimination of sampling error. Because it is the endoscopist's perception of the image that dictates the intervention in Barrett's esophagus and early-stage adenocarcinoma, authors review the cutting edge technology in endoscopic imaging.

This issue was designed for the provider who encounters patients with complex gastroesophageal reflux disease such as those with end-stage lung disease, atypical symptoms, morbid obesity, and Barrett's esophagus with dysplasia. With the recent introduction of endolumenal therapies for Barrett's esophagus and dysplasia (radiofrequency ablation, cryoablation, endoscopic resection, and endoscopic submucosal resection), the rationale for esophageal preservation is addressed and an algorithm for therapy and surveillance is presented.

Novel approaches to esophageal motility disorders are introduced and reviewed. The approach and outcomes of transoral stapling of Zenker's diverticulum, a very significant contribution to the treatment of cricopharyngeal achalasia in the last decade, are covered in detail. The introduction of the endoscopic myotomy for the treatment of achalasia highlights the importance of the flexible endoscope in the future of esophageal surgery and takes minimally invasive surgery to a whole new realm: Incisionless. Staying with the endoscopic theme, the cutting edge in the management of esophageal perforation is covered in detail and

Thorac Surg Clin 21 (2011) ix–xi
doi:10.1016/j.thorsurg.2011.09.002
1547-4127/11/$ – see front matter © 2011 Elsevier Inc. All rights reserved.

provides readers with a treatment algorithm that is practical and evidence based.

I am extremely grateful to the contributing authors for their thoughtful and experience-based insights into the most challenging corners of benign esophageal diseases and believe that this issue of *Thoracic Surgery Clinics* will be drawn upon for "advice" for years to come. I would like to thank the Consulting Editor of *Thoracic Surgery Clinics*, Mark K. Ferguson, MD for his vision and expertise and Barbara Cohen-Kligerman from Elsevier, who was instrumental in bringing this work to the "finish line."

Blair A. Jobe, MD
Division of Thoracic and Foregut Surgery
Department of Cardiothoracic Surgery
University of Pittsburgh Medical Center
5200 Centre Avenue, Suite 715
Pittsburgh, PA 15232, USA

E-mail address:
jobeba@upmc.edu

Dedication

This issue is dedicated to Tom R. DeMeester for his example and guidance. He built the road upon which we travel forward.

The Cutting Edge in Esophageal Physiology Testing: Equipment, Uses, and Analysis

Thomas J. Watson, MD

KEYWORDS

- Esophageal physiology • Esophageal diagnostics
- High-resolution manometry
- Esophageal pressure topography
- Multichannel intraluminal impedance
- Ambulatory pH monitoring

Benign esophageal diseases consist of a spectrum of disorders of varying causes and clinical manifestations. The esophageal surgeon must be well versed in esophageal anatomy, physiology, and pathologic conditions to understand the genesis of a patients' symptoms and to provide a rationale for therapy. The relationship between symptoms and objective findings, however, is often not clear. This observation may result, at least in part, from the fact that the diagnostic tools used to assess foregut physiology historically have been fairly crude, imperfect, and limited in scope. In recent years, however, evolutionary technologies have advanced the understanding of both normal and abnormal foregut structure and function.

The landscape of esophageal diagnostics began to change in the 1990s with the introduction of 3 technologies: high-resolution manometry (HRM), multichannel intraluminal impedance (MII) testing, and the Bravo pH monitoring system (Given Imaging, Duluth, GA, USA). The first and last technologies represent replacements for previously existing modalities, whereas the second represents a whole new diagnostic paradigm in the foregut arena. Taken together, the 3 technologies have dramatically changed the way in which esophageal physiology is assessed. An understanding of these technologies, therefore, is imperative for the practicing esophageal surgeon because their interpretation may have significant implications relative to surgical decision making.

HRM AND ESOPHAGEAL PRESSURE TOPOGRAPHY

The introduction of HRM into clinical practice in 2000, along with the development of sophisticated algorithms to display the expanded data set as esophageal pressure topography plots, has transformed conventional esophageal manometry from an analysis of wave tracings to an image-based paradigm assisted with color enhancements (**Fig. 1**). Just as high-definition television has made standard-definition broadcasting seem antiquated, HRM has made conventional manometry (CM) seem obsolete.

High-resolution esophageal pressure topography (HREPT) is not synonymous with HRM. HRM merely implies that manometry is performed with multiple closely spaced sensors, typically at 1-cm intervals. Pressure sensors are spaced in such close proximity to each other that, by interpolating between sensors, intraluminal pressure is represented as a pressure continuum from the pharynx to the stomach. Pressure topography, on the other hand, refers to the manner in which

Department of Surgery, University of Rochester School of Medicine and Dentistry, 601 Elmwood Avenue, Box Surgery, Rochester, NY 14642, USA
E-mail address: Thomas_Watson@urmc.rochester.edu

Thorac Surg Clin 21 (2011) 449–463
doi:10.1016/j.thorsurg.2011.08.003
1547-4127/11/$ – see front matter © 2011 Elsevier Inc. All rights reserved.

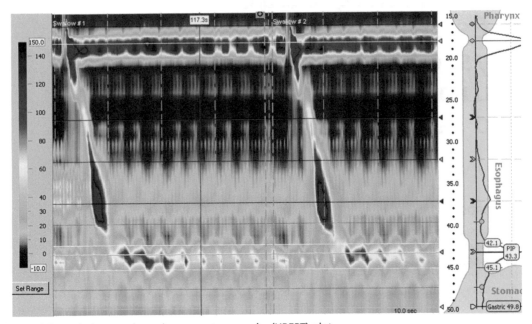

Fig. 1. High-resolution esophageal pressure topography (HREPT) plot.

manometric data are displayed and analyzed. First described by Clouse,[1] HREPT consists of isobaric contour plots with pressures depicted using color, 3-dimensional elevation, or both. Time is placed on the x-axis and sensor position along the pharynx/esophagus/esophagogastric junction/stomach along the y-axis. Thus, although HRM and HREPT are not synonymous, HRM is necessary to create HREPT.

Equipment and Technique

The HRM catheter (Given Imaging, Duluth, GA, USA) is 4.2 mm in diameter and consists of 36 solid-state circumferential sensors spaced at 1-cm increments (**Fig. 2**). The equipment uses pressure transduction technology (TactArray, Given Imaging, Duluth, GA, USA) that allows each sensor to detect pressure over a length of 2.5 mm in 12 radially dispersed sectors. The sector pressures are averaged, making each of the 36 sensors a circumferential pressure detector. The solid-state frequency response characteristics of each sensing element can capture pressure changes

in excess of 6000 mm Hg/s and accurate to within 1 mm Hg of atmospheric pressure. The data acquisition frequency is 35 Hz for each sensor. The data are then analyzed using ManoView (Given Imaging, Duluth, GA, USA) analysis software.

The procedure is performed in the author's laboratory by a trained esophageal laboratory nurse in conjunction with an esophageal fellow. Patients are instructed to take in nothing by mouth for at least 6 hours before the examination. The patient's nasal passages are topically anesthetized and the catheter is passed transnasally by the nurse. The catheter is positioned to allow analysis of the deglutitive response from the hypopharynx to the stomach with a minimum of 4 intragastric sensors. Only 1 positioning of the catheter is necessary, unlike CM whereby the catheter must be incrementally withdrawn during analysis of the lower esophageal sphincter (LES) and repositioned to assess esophageal body function. The catheter is then taped to the nose.

The fellow is responsible for the conduct of the study, including the confirmation of accurate catheter placement spanning the upper esophageal sphincter (UES) and the LES, appropriate patient swallowing and timing between swallows, concurrent study interpretation to assure quality control, and troubleshooting. Errors in catheter positioning, function, or study conduct can be recognized by typical HREPT patterns (**Figs. 3–6**). At the start of the procedure, the transducers are calibrated to 0 and 100 mm Hg using externally applied pressure. Patients are placed in the supine

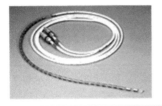

Fig. 2. HRM catheter.

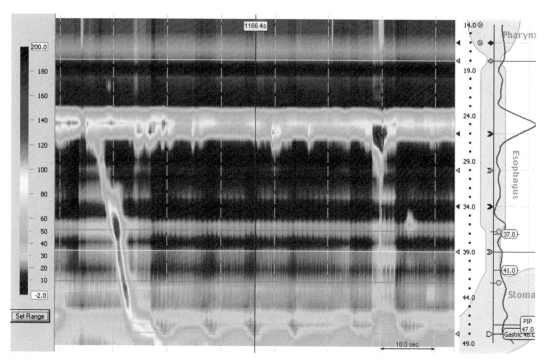

Fig. 3. A poorly positioned HRM catheter. The catheter sensors are too proximal to allow full analysis of the esophagogastric junction.

position. Once patients have accommodated to the catheter, data acquisition begins with a 30-second swallow-free period to allow assessment of the basal pressure and length characteristics of the UES and LES (the landmark frame). The resting pressure of the LES is determined at the respiratory pressure inversion point (PIP), the level at which pressures transition from a positive deflection (intra-abdominal) to a negative deflection (intrathoracic) with inspiration (**Fig. 7**). As

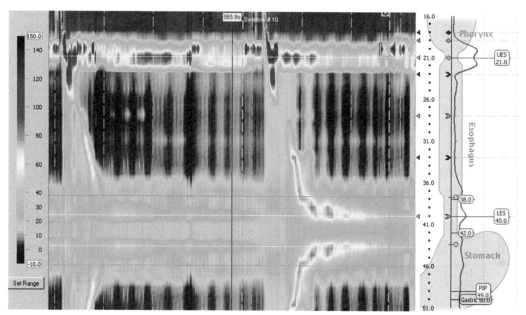

Fig. 4. HRM catheter that is doubled back on itself, leading to a butterfly effect in the plot. PIP, pressure inversion point.

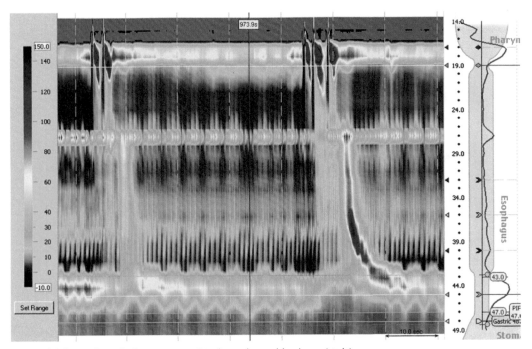

Fig. 5. Multiple swallows before a transmitted esophageal body peristaltic wave.

with CM, HRM studies then consist of a series of water swallows, generally 10 consecutive swallows of 5 mL of water at least 25 seconds apart. Although alternative postures or swallowed substances may be used, the normal values have been based on these conventions.

Analysis

The landmark frame is assessed to obtain baseline reference values for the UES and LES. The LES analysis consists of a resting pressure as well as total and abdominal lengths. Abdominal length is

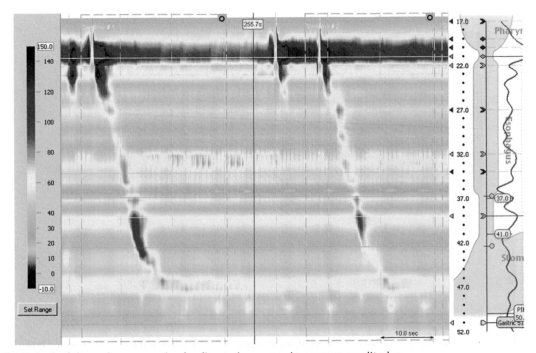

Fig. 6. Lack of thermal compensation leading to inaccuracy in pressure amplitudes.

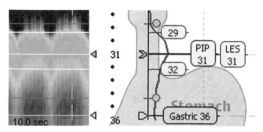

Fig. 7. The landmark frame demonstrating LES upper and lower borders, PIP, and resting pressure.

defined as the portion from the bottom of the sphincter to the PIP. A hiatal hernia is evidenced by the presence of 2 distal high-pressure zones.

The wet swallows are then analyzed to assess UES contraction, UES relaxation, esophageal body peristaltic function, and LES relaxation. Measurements of the LES are made by dragging the corresponding icons (LES upper border, LES lower border, PIP) up or down the right side of the screen in the pressure profile to the appropriate level.

The analysis software contains an interpretive aid called the isobaric contour tool. This function allows boundaries to be drawn around any designated pressure value. Setting such a boundary at 15 mm Hg, for instance, results in the creation of boundary lines demonstrating a cut-off between

pressures more than and less than 15 mm Hg. If, in analyzing esophagogastric junction (EGJ) relaxation during wet swallows, the boundary lines do not come together signifying a break in the isobaric contour, the EGJ pressure never drops less than 15 mm Hg (the upper limit for normal EGJ relaxation pressure in the author's laboratory) and EGJ relaxation is incomplete (**Fig. 8**). Similarly, the boundary can be set at 20 mm Hg to determine interrupted esophageal body contractions (when the wave amplitudes decreases less than this value).

Several new terms have arisen along with the introduction of HRM that are important for the esophagologist to understand. These terms, as defined by the Chicago Classification of HREPT,[2] are as follows:

1. Four-second integrated relaxation pressure (4-second IRP; millimeters of mercury): The mean value of the esophagogastric junction (EGJ) pressure, measured by a contiguous or noncontiguous window of 4 seconds of relaxation in the 10-second window following deglutitive UES relaxation, using the difference between the electronic equivalent of a sleeve sensor and gastric channels (**Fig. 9**). This value is commonly used as the measure of EGJ relaxation. An elevated 4-second IRP (more than 15 mm Hg in the author's laboratory) suggests

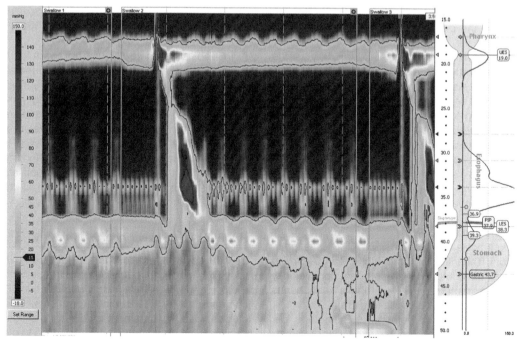

Fig. 8. A poorly relaxing LES during a wet swallow. Note that the isobaric contour lines denoting a pressure of 15 mm Hg never converge, signifying a lack of relaxation.

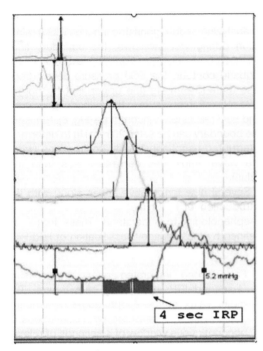

Fig. 9. Four-second IRP.

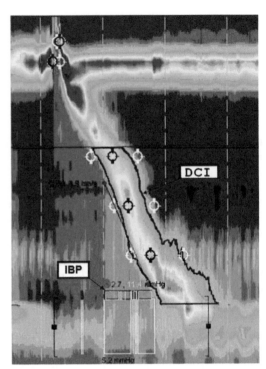

Fig. 10. The DCI and intrabolus pressure (IBP).

impaired deglutitive EGJ relaxation as seen in typical achalasia or other causes of esophageal outflow obstruction.

2. Distal contractile integral (DCI; millimeters of mercury × seconds × centimeters): The integrated value of pressures more than 20 mm Hg in the distal esophagus. The time boundaries are within the span of the swallow being analyzed. The distal boundary is the upper border of the LES, whereas the proximal boundary is the pressure nadir (P) between the first and second esophageal segments (corresponding to the transition zone between striated and smooth esophageal muscle). The DCI represents contraction amplitude × duration × length (**Fig. 10**), and the normal range is 500 to 4300 mm Hg × s × cm in the author's laboratory. An elevated DCI can be seen with hypercontractility of the esophagus, whereas a low DCI signifies hypoperistalsis, such as seen with scleroderma.

3. Contractile deceleration point (CDP; time, position): The inflection point along the 30-mm Hg isobaric contour where propagation velocity slows demarcating the tubular esophagus from the phrenic ampulla (**Fig. 11**).

4. Contractile front velocity (centimeters per second): The slope of the tangent approximating the 30-mm Hg isobaric contour between the P and the CDP (see **Fig. 11**).

5. Distal latency (seconds): The interval between UES relaxation and the CDP (**Fig. 12**). A latency period less than 4.5 seconds signifies rapid propagation of an esophageal wave.

6. Peristaltic breaks (centimeters): Gaps in the 20-mm Hg isobaric contour of the peristaltic contraction between the UES and the EGJ measured in axial length.

7. Intrabolus pressure (IBP): The mean of the maximum pressures generated within the esophageal bolus (preceding the esophageal contractile wave) during a 3-second period restricted to exclude regions of significant pressure gradient (>2 mm Hg) and taken relative to atmospheric pressure (see **Fig. 10**). The IBP may be elevated when there is significant resistance to esophageal outflow, such as in achalasia, paraesophageal hernia, or after fundoplication.

HRM Versus Conventional Manometry

Several advantages exist for HREPT compared with CM, although published reports analyzing the comparison are few. A trial published in 2000 compared CM with HRM in 212 patients.[1] The 2 studies were in agreement in 88% of the cases. Conventional manometry, however, failed to diagnose achalasia in 6 of 36 patients detected by HRM. In addition, CM failed to recognize 12

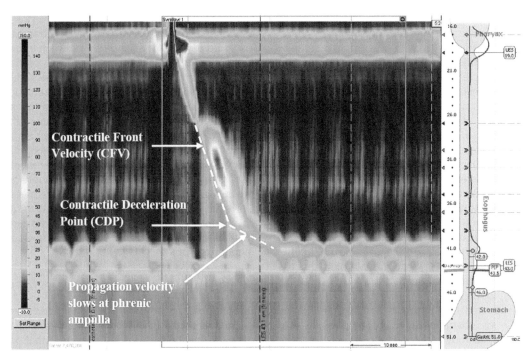

Fig. 11. Contractile front velocity and CDP.

patients with incomplete LES relaxation identified with HRM. An additional observation was that HRM better identified the position of the LES relative to the hiatus in patients with a hiatal hernia.

The position of the LES is important when transnasal pH monitoring is performed and the pH electrode is placed relative to the upper border of the LES. These data suggest that HRM is superior to

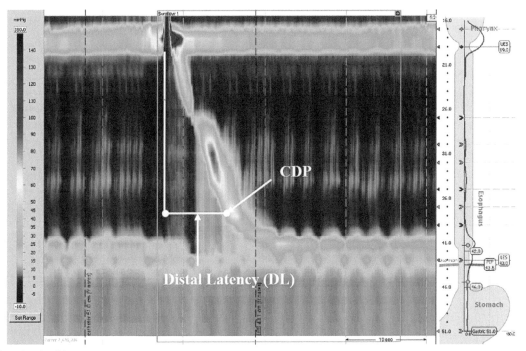

Fig. 12. Distal latency.

CM, particularly relative to the identification of poor LES relaxation and LES position.

Another advantage of HRM is that the catheter can be positioned once for a study, unlike CM when multiple repositionings and sequential withdrawal are necessary. The time to perform a study, therefore, is shorter with less patient discomfort. Data from the author's laboratory reveal that HRM studies, on average, required 8.1 minutes to complete, whereas CM typically lasted 24.4 minutes.[3] Once completed, the HRM studies are easier to interpret. The HREPT plots are also quickly analyzed and intuitive. Distinct diagnoses, such as normal esophageal peristalsis (**Fig. 13**), the presence of a hiatal hernia (**Fig. 14**), typical achalasia (**Fig. 15**), nutcracker esophagus (**Fig. 16**), and diffuse esophageal spasm (**Fig. 17**), commonly yield easily recognizable plots that the interpreter can readily detect.

The introduction of HRM has allowed more sophisticated data analysis and has led to the ability to characterize EGJ competence and esophageal body peristaltic function in ways never previously possible. Kahrilas, Pandolfino, and associates[4] from Northwestern University used HRM/HREPT to assess functional LES and crural diaphragm contributions to the pathogenesis of gastroesophageal reflux disease (GERD). They found LES-crural diaphragm separation to be one of the factors responsible for the early stages of GERD. In a separate publication, the Northwestern group used HRM/HREPT to classify esophageal motility disorders in 400 patients.[5] They were able to distinguish between rapidly propagated contractions (spasm) and compartmentalized pressurization. With this differentiation, they determined spastic disorders (diffuse esophageal spasm, vigorous achalasia, and spastic nutcracker) to be rare. In a third publication, they subclassified achalasia into 3 distinct types, all characterized by impaired EGJ relaxation and esophageal body aperistalsis, but differentiated from one another by the degree of esophageal pressurization (**Box 1**).[6] The author's group at the University of Rochester recently described and categorized atypical variants of achalasia using HRM, finding them more common than previously recognized (**Box 2**).[7]

MULTICHANNEL INTRALUMINAL IMPEDANCE

Esophageal manometry, whether performed by conventional or high-resolution techniques, measures esophageal luminal pressures that drive bolus transit. A limitation of manometry is that bolus movement is not directly assessed. The correlation between effective peristalsis and bolus clearance, however, is only moderate; patients may complain of dysphagia while having normal peristaltic function as assessed by manometry. Similarly, significant peristaltic dysfunction may be seen in asymptomatic patients with normal

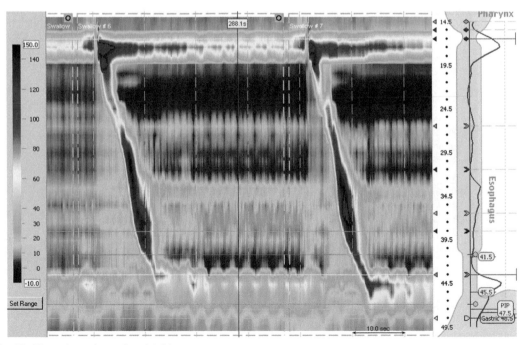

Fig. 13. Normal esophageal peristalsis.

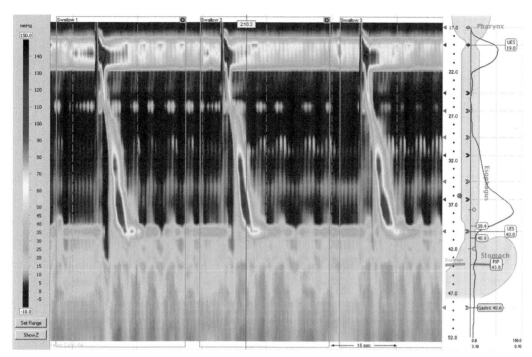

Fig. 14. Hiatal hernia noted by the presence of 2 EGJ high-pressure zones and a short or absent LES length.

bolus transit. The ability to assess bolus movement, therefore, holds appeal for the evaluation of patients with dysphagia. Although videofluoroscopy with barium swallows has been used for this purpose, exposure to radiation is necessary, and temporal correlation to manometric findings can pose a challenge. Impedance monitoring is a newer, catheter-based modality

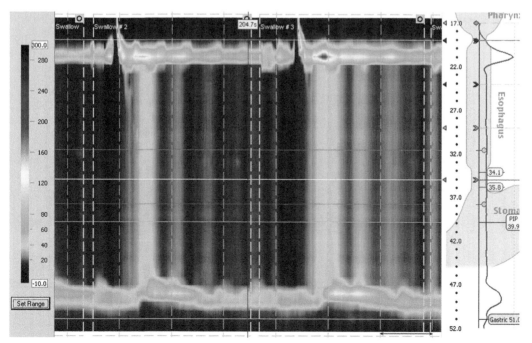

Fig. 15. Achalasia characterized by a hypertensive, poorly relaxing LES, esophageal body aperistalsis, and pressurization.

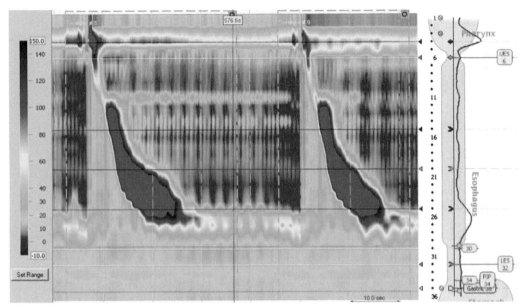

Fig. 16. Nutcracker esophagus characterized by peristaltic waves with an amplitude more than 180 mm Hg or DCI more than 5000 mm Hg × seconds × centimeters.

that was developed to assess transit within the esophagus, thus, facilitating detection of antegrade bolus movement on swallowing or retrograde movement of gastric contents when refluxed. Impedance monitoring has utility in assessment of patients with dysphagia and esophageal motility disorders as well as in the evaluation of GERD.

Impedance is the ratio of voltage to current and is a measure of the electrical conductivity of a hollow organ and its contents. Impedance is inversely proportional to the electrical conductivity

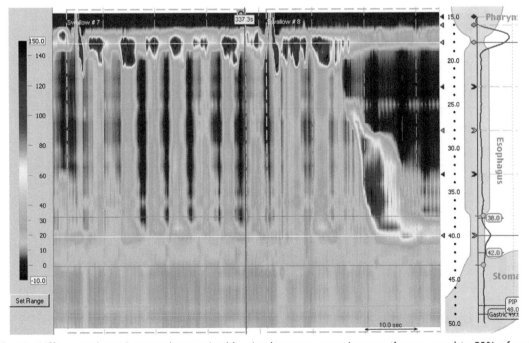

Fig. 17. Diffuse esophageal spasm characterized by simultaneous waves in more than or equal to 20% of wet swallows, intermittent peristaltic waves, and prolonged contractions in the distal esophagus (>6 seconds).

Box 1
Subclassification of achalasia based on HRM findings

Type I (classic): Achalasia with minimal compression ($\leq$30 mm Hg)

Type II: Achalasia with compression (>30 mm Hg in at least 2 wet swallows)

Type III: Achalasia with spasm (in at least 2 wet swallows)

(*Data from* Pandolfino JE, Kwiatek MA, Nealis T, et al. Achalasia: a new clinically relevant classification by high-resolution manometry. Gastroenterology 2008; 135:1526–33.)

---

of the luminal contents and the cross-sectional area of the lumen. Air has low electrical conductivity and, therefore, high impedance. Saliva, food, and gastric juice cause a decrease in impedance because of their high conductivity. Luminal dilation leads to decreased impedance, whereas luminal contraction causes increased impedance.

Esophageal impedance monitoring has been validated as an appropriate method for the assessment of the transit of a swallowed bolus through the esophagus by comparison with cineradiographic images.[8] Bolus entry, movement, and exit can be detected by impedance changes in the appropriate segments. The performance of an impedance-based esophageal transit study is similar to standard manometry. Several catheter configurations are commercially available, with the impedance electrodes typically placed 2 cm apart. The catheter is passed transnasally and positioned appropriately within the esophagus. A manometry study is typically performed before or concurrent with the impedance study. Combined impedance-manometry catheters are also commercially available. The catheter is taped to the nose and 10 swallows of 5-mL saline boluses

---

Box 2
Classification of variant achalasia

Type I: Abnormal LES with normal/hypertensive peristalsis

Type II: Abnormal/borderline LES with spastic or partially spastic contractile waves

Type III: Borderline/normal LES and aperistalsis with occasional short segment peristalsis

(*From* Galey KM, Wilshire CL, Niebisch S, et al. Atypical variants of classic achalasia are common and currently under-recognized: a study of prevalence and clinical features. J Am Coll Surg 2011;213:155–63; with permission.)

---

are given. The resultant tracings are analyzed for the passage of air and fluid. Bolus entry is determined by a greater than or equal to 50% decrease in impedance from baseline relative to nadir, whereas bolus exit is determined by a greater than or equal to 50% recovery from nadir to baseline.

For impedance monitoring to be clinically useful in the evaluation of esophageal motility disorders, it has to provide reliable and meaningful information on bolus transit. This requirement seems to have been met based on validation studies comparing impedance assessment with videofluoroscopy. Secondly, impedance testing needs to provide additional relevant information compared with HRM. The combination of impedance testing and HRM needs to be more clinically useful than HRM alone. This second requirement has yet to be met. The thresholds for determining normal and abnormal bolus transit, and their correlation with the presence or absence of dysphagia, are poorly defined and unreliable at present. Thus, it is unlikely that impedance testing will replace videofluoroscopy in the assessment of patients with dysphagia.

High-Resolution Impedance Manometry

A catheter combining both HRM and high-resolution impedance was recently introduced (Given Imaging, Duluth, GA, USA). The catheter allows simultaneous assessment of HRM tracings and bolus clearance as assessed by impedance monitoring (**Fig. 18**A and B) displayed in a color format. The HRM plots are the same as for standard HRM. Bolus presence is denoted by a superimposed purple color. Bolus clearance is classified as either complete or incomplete. Although the author has been using this technology, particularly in the evaluation of patients with dysphagia, its clinical value relative to other available modalities, including HRM alone, has yet to be determined.

MII-pH Monitoring

Traditional ambulatory esophageal pH monitoring is limited by the fact that it works by detection of acidic liquid less than a pH of 4 at a specific point within the esophageal lumen; the volume, height, and chemical composition of the refluxate are not discernible. The addition of MII to standard pH monitoring allows the detection not only of esophageal acid but also the presence of nonacidic or weakly acidic reflux events at multiple levels and the direction of bolus movement within the esophagus.

An MII catheter was designed with multiple electrodes placed at 2-cm increments to allow

A   B

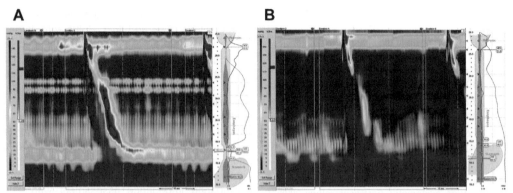

Fig. 18. (*A*) Combined HRM high-resolution impedance tracings demonstrating complete bolus clearance. The purple coloration denotes the presence of a liquid bolus within the esophagus. The bolus is cleared in front of the contractile wave. (*B*) Combined HRM high-resolution impedance tracings demonstrating incomplete bolus clearance. Note that liquid remains within the esophageal body after passage of the contractile wave.

assessment of impedance at 3, 5, 7, 9, 15, and 17 cm from the distal tip. The multiple electrodes permit detection of the direction and velocity of bolus transport through the esophagus. An extremely low electric current of 0.00025 μW is transmitted across the electrodes at a frequency of 1 to 2 kHz and limited to 8 μA, less than the threshold for stimulation of nerves, muscles, and the cardiac conduction system. The author uses a catheter that also has pH sensors 5 cm and 20 cm from the distal tip.

Esophageal manometry is a prerequisite to MII-pH monitoring to determine the position of the LES relative to the nares. After the MII-pH catheter is passed transnasally and appropriately positioned within the esophagus, patients are instructed on the appropriate diet and told to keep a diary of the time and content of meals, the beginning and end of recumbency at night, and the time/type of symptoms experienced. After a 24-hour period, patients return the data logger and the diary, the data are uploaded, and analysis is performed using dedicated software (Sleuth, Sandhill Scientific, Highlands Ranch, CO, USA). Despite the fact that the analysis is automated, manual review of the tracings is also required to detect measurement artifacts, missed reflux events, or swallowed boluses interpreted by the software as reflux episodes (**Fig. 19**).

The addition of MII to pH monitoring has led to new classifications of gastroesophageal reflux events based on the content of the refluxate (liquid, gas, or mixed) and the degree of acidity (acidic, weakly acidic, or nonacidic). A consensus panel classified reflux events with a pH less than 4 as acidic, those with a pH between 4 and 7 as weakly acidic, and those with a pH greater than 7 as nonacidic.[9]

Normal values for MII-pH monitoring performed off of acid-suppressive therapy were established in a multi-institutional study of 60 healthy, adult volunteers.[10] In asymptomatic individuals, most reflux events were acidic, with nonacidic events clustered in the postprandial periods. In addition, only 37% of acidic or nonacidic reflux events detected at the distal sensor (5 cm more than the LES) reached the proximal sensor (15 cm more than the LES). Additional studies have revealed that the addition of acid-suppressive therapy does not reduce the number of reflux events but merely converts them to a more neutral pH.[11]

Combined MII-pH monitoring has been used in several clinical circumstances. Traditionally, patients with suspected GERD have been given an empiric trial of acid-suppressive therapy with a proton pump inhibitor (PPI) or H2-receptor antagonist. For those patients whose symptoms respond, the diagnosis of GERD is assumed and therapy is continued. Nonresponders may be offered pH monitoring while on therapy to assess whether symptoms are temporally correlated to reflux events or after the discontinuation of PPI therapy for at least 7 days to assess excessive esophageal acid exposure. This approach ignores the potential for nonacidic or weakly acidic reflux events. Because combined MII-pH monitoring performed on PPI therapy allows the detection of these other reflux events, the technology can be used to differentiate patients into those having symptoms associated with ongoing acid reflux (for whom increased acid suppression may be an option), symptoms associated with non–acid reflux (suggesting the need for an antireflux operation or endoscopic augmentation of the LES), or symptoms not associated with any type of reflux (suggesting a non-GERD cause). Using this

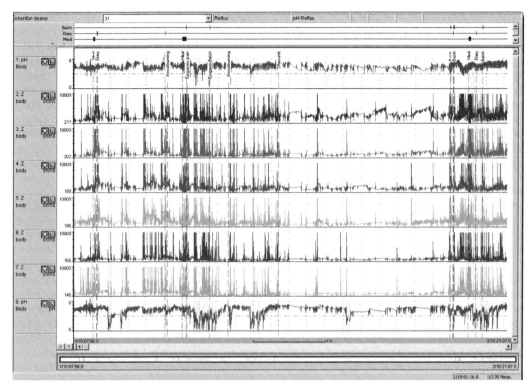

Fig. 19. Excessive gastroesophageal reflux as detected on MII-pH monitoring.

approach, patients with persistent symptoms while on PPI therapy have been referred for fundoplication with a high likelihood of a successful symptomatic outcome.[12] Such a diagnostic and treatment paradigm may be particularly useful in patients with various extraesophageal manifestations of GERD because the diagnostic yield of traditional pH monitoring performed while off of acid-suppressive therapy is less compared with patients presenting with typical reflux symptoms of heartburn and regurgitation.

Bravo pH Monitoring System

Ambulatory esophageal pH monitoring has long been considered the gold standard for the determination of the presence of pathologic esophageal acid exposure. Traditional monitoring involves transnasal placement of an antimony or glass pH electrode 5 cm above the manometrically determined upper border of the LES and a study duration of 24 hours. This technique suffers from the need for a transnasal catheter for an extended period of time and the resultant patient discomfort, dissatisfaction, and noncompliance. Some patients simply cannot tolerate catheter placement at all or for the 24-hour time period, resulting in a considerable failure rate in obtaining meaningful results.

The Bravo pH monitoring system permits the wireless transmission of esophageal pH data, improving patient compliance and facilitating a longer period of monitoring. As a result of these advantages, the Bravo system has replaced traditional catheter-based pH monitoring at many centers in most cases.

The Bravo capsule measures 6.0 mm × 5.5 mm × 25.0 mm (**Fig. 20**A) and consists of antimony pH and reference electrodes at the distal tip, an internal battery, and a radio transmitter. The pH capsule sends data to an external receiver worn by patients during the study period (see **Fig. 20**B). Data are transmitted at 433 MHz, an unregulated band, and data security is maintained

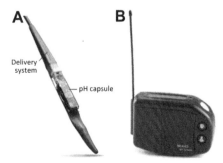

Fig. 20. (A) Bravo capsule and introducer system. (B) External receiver.

by digital transmission of a unique code every 12 seconds, along with 2 pH data points obtained at 6-second sampling intervals. Before placement, the capsule is calibrated by submersion in buffer solutions at pH 7.01 and 1.07.

In the author's facility, the capsule is placed at the time of flexible upper endoscopy, although it may also be placed transnasally using manometrically determined landmarks. The location of the EGJ is noted relative to the incisors and is determined by the upper limit of the gastric rugal folds. The Bravo capsule is introduced transorally via its delivery system, which contains a sheath at the tip to protect the capsule and facilitate passage through the mouth and pharynx. The capsule is positioned 6 cm above the EGJ, using the depth markings along the shaft. The endoscope is reinserted so that the capsule can be deployed under direct endoscopic visualization. The capsule contains a well measuring 4.0 mm in diameter and 3.5 mm in depth into which the esophageal mucosa is suctioned. Care should be taken to avoid the placement of excess lubricant in the vicinity of the well because unsuccessful mucosal capture may result. Suction is applied to the capsule using the supplied suction unit, which is

capable of providing 600 mm Hg of vacuum pressure. Successful mucosal capture is assumed when the suction pressure is more than 510 mm Hg for at least 30 seconds. The activation button on the delivery system is pressed, releasing a spring-loaded pin through the well tangential to the esophageal axis, securing the esophageal mucosa within the well. The activation button is then rotated 90°clockwise and re-extended, releasing the capsule from the delivery system, which is then withdrawn. Endoscopy confirms appropriate capture of the esophageal mucosa within the capsule.

Patients are instructed on the appropriate use of the receiver, which they typically wear on their waist, and are told to maintain a diary of symptoms, meals, and time of recumbence. Data typically are collected for 48 hours, as compared with the standard of 24 hours for conventional catheter-based pH monitoring. Many patients report a foreign body sensation within their esophagus as long as the capsule is present, although this is generally well tolerated. Patients return the external receiver after the study period. The capsule typically sloughs within 5 to 7 days. The author avoids fundoplication within the first

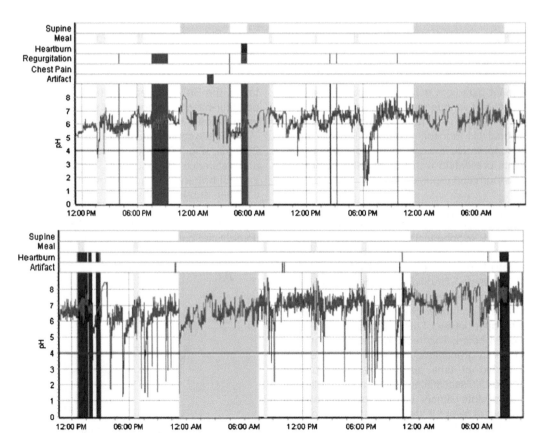

Fig. 21. Bravo pH tracings.

10 to 14 days of a Bravo study for fear that the capsule may still be present within the esophagus and result in a mucosal laceration if an esophageal bougie is passed during surgery. The manufacturer also states that magnetic resonance imaging is contraindicated within 30 days of a Bravo study for fear that the capsule may still reside somewhere along the gastrointestinal tract.

Data analysis is accomplished with automated software after entry of symptoms, the timing of meals, and the upright and supine time periods (**Fig. 21**). A summary of the pH data contains the parameters measured for traditional catheter-based pH monitoring, including the total time and percentage time pH less than 4, the longest reflux episode with pH less than 4, the total number of reflux episodes, the number of episodes with pH less than 4 for greater than 5 minutes, the total duration of pH recording, the total time and percentage time upright and supine, the DeMeester score for each 24-hour time period, and the aggregate score for 48 hours. Normal values for esophageal acid exposure have been derived and are similar to the values seen with traditional catheter-based pH monitoring.[13] Although patients generally tolerate Bravo pH monitoring quite well, disadvantages include the need for endoscopy, the potential for significant chest pain, and the possibility of early capsule dislodgement invalidating the study.

SUMMARY

Advancements in foregut diagnostic technologies have led to improvements in the esophagologist's ability to accurately diagnose and classify esophageal pathophysiology and increased patient satisfaction and compliance in undergoing testing. Consistent with the adage that diagnosis should precede treatment, the esophageal surgeon's ability to bring about a successful outcome is dependent on the proper application and interpretation of these diagnostic modalities. Because symptoms suggestive of foregut pathologic conditions are often nonspecific and readily confused with complaints having their genesis in nonforegut causes, the ability to reliably and consistently differentiate foregut disorders from other potential contributors is an essential ingredient in assuring appropriate therapy and predicting success. With ongoing study and refinement, the recently introduced esophageal physiologic studies will inevitably continue to improve and additional technologies will continue to emerge. The physician or surgeon treating esophageal disorders is well advised to keep abreast of ongoing advancements and to implement them, as appropriate, into their diagnostic armamentarium.

REFERENCES

1. Clouse RE, Staiano A, Alrakawi A, et al. Application of topographical methods to clinical esophageal manometry. Am J Gastroenterol 2000;95:2720–30.
2. Kahrilas PJ, Ghosh SK, Pandolfino JE. Esophageal motility disorders in terms of pressure topography: the Chicago Classification. J Clin Gastroenterol 2008;42:627–35.
3. Salvador R, Dubecz A, Polomsky M, et al. A new era in esophageal diagnostics: the image-based paradigm of high-resolution manometry. J Am Coll Surg 2009;208:1035–44.
4. Pandolfino JE, Kim H, Ghosh SK, et al. High-resolution manometry of the EGJ: an analysis of crural diaphragm function in GERD. Am J Gastroenterol 2007; 102:1056–63.
5. Pandolfino JE, Ghosh SK, Rice J, et al. Classifying esophageal motility by pressure topography characteristics: a study of 400 patients and 75 controls. Am J Gastroenterol 2008;103:27–37.
6. Pandolfino JE, Kwiatek MA, Nealis T, et al. Achalasia: a new clinically relevant classification by high-resolution manometry. Gastroenterology 2008; 135:1526–33.
7. Galey KM, Wilshire CL, Niebisch S, et al. Atypical variants of classic achalasia are common and currently under-recognized: a study of prevalence and clinical features. J Am Coll Surg 2011;213: 155–63.
8. Imam H, Shay S, Ali A, et al. Bolus transit patterns in healthy subjects: a study using simultaneous impedance monitoring, videoesophagram, and esophageal manometry. Am J Physiol Gastrointest Liver Physiol 2005;288:G1000–6.
9. Sifrim D, Castell DO, Dent J, et al. Gastroesophageal reflux monitoring: review and consensus report on detection and definitions of acid, non-acid and gas reflux. Gut 2004;53:1024–31.
10. Shay SS, Tutuian R, Sifrim D, et al. Twenty-four hour ambulatory simultaneous impedance and pH monitoring: a multicenter report of normal values from 60 healthy volunteers. Am J Gastroenterol 2004;99: 1037–43.
11. Tamhankar A, Peters JH, Portale G, et al. Omeprazole does not reduce gastroesophageal reflux: new insights using multichannel intraluminal impedance technology. J Gastrointest Surg 2004;8: 888–96.
12. Mainie I, Tutuian R, Agrawal A, et al. Combined multichannel intraluminal impedance-pH monitoring to select patients with persistent gastro-oesophageal reflux for laparoscopic Nissen fundoplication. Br J Surg 2006;93:1483–7.
13. Pandolfino JE, Richter JE, Ours T, et al. Ambulatory esophageal pH monitoring using a wireless system. Am J Gastroenterol 2003;98:740–9.

High-Resolution Manometry: An Atlas of Esophageal Motility Disorders and Findings of GERD Using Esophageal Pressure Topography

John E. Pandolfino, MD[a],*, Sabine Roman, MD, PhD[b]

KEYWORDS

- High-resolution manometry
- Esophageal pressure topography
- Gastroesophageal reflux disease • Dysphagia

High-resolution manometry (HRM), in and of itself, is an adaptation of conventional manometric hardware that basically employs an increased number of pressure sensors spaced closely together. The data generated by HRM would therefore be displayed as a tracing format similar to what would be used for conventional manometric interpretation. The real advance in terms of manometry is primarily focused on the analysis techniques that were derived to optimize the information from high-resolution manometry. To better visualize the data, Clouse and Staino[1] incorporated a process of interpolation or averaging between sensors to display the information in the form of seamless isobaric color regions on esophageal pressure topography plots (EPT) (**Fig. 1**). The EPT or "Clouse plots" have the capacity to convert manometric information into distinct patterns that illustrate the physiology of contractile coordination and the mechanics associated with bolus transit. In addition, Hebbard's group also deserve special mention in any discussion on HRM, as they were responsible for developing one of the first analysis software packages focused on EPT. This software was subsequently used to define subtle peristaltic defects important in bolus transit that were missed with conventional manometry.[2]

Although this technique was reserved primarily for research centers, it has now become widely available and currently is moving into mainstream clinical practice. Fortunately, there has been a substantial amount of work that has adapted the concepts of the classification scheme used in conventional manometry into a new classification for EPT that incorporates the added detail and accuracy of this new analysis technique. This work has resulted in a new classification scheme and the development of new measurements

This work was supported by R01 DK079902 (JEP) from the Public Health Service.
Conflict of Interest: John E. Pandolfino [Given Imaging (Consulting, Educational)] Sabine Roman [Given Imaging].
[a] Department of Medicine, Feinberg School of Medicine, Northwestern University, 676 St Clair Street, Suite 1400, Chicago, IL 60611-2951, USA
[b] Digestive Physiology, Edouard Herriot Hospital, Hospices Civils de Lyon, Université Claude Bernard Lyon I, Lyon, France
* Corresponding author.
E-mail address: j-pandolfino@northwestern.edu

Thorac Surg Clin 21 (2011) 465–475
doi:10.1016/j.thorsurg.2011.08.007

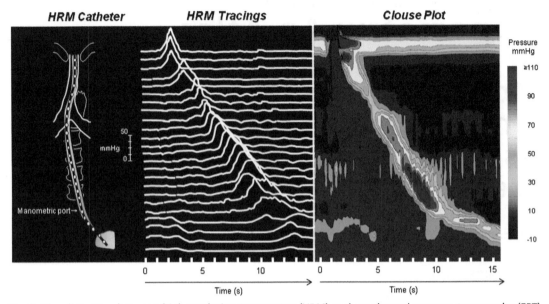

Fig. 1. The distinction between high-resolution manometry (HRM) and esophageal pressure topography (EPT). The HRM catheter consists of 21 to 36 closely spaced pressure sensors. The position of pressure sensors in the esophagus is indicated in the anatomic drawing on the left. In the middle panel, the data from HRM recordings are displayed as tracings for each pressure sensor similar to conventional manometry. EPT is illustrated on the right. EPT is distinct from HRM in that it is purely a data analysis method whereas HRM is a data acquisition method. The Clouse plots (EPT plots) are derived from the data acquired from HRM and are displayed using a color code to describe peristaltic amplitude in a space-time continuum. A technique of interpolating between the recording sensors allows one to obtain a seamless representation of the pressure activity through the entire swallow. Note the tremendously enhanced detail provided by the Clouse plot, especially in the area of the esophagogastric junction.

derived specifically for EPT that focus heavily on pattern recognition of contractile and bolus pressurization patterns. Thus, EPT is more akin to an imaging technique as opposed to a data output stream displayed over time.

The goal of this article is to provide an atlas of esophageal motility disorders focused on dysphagia and gastroesophageal reflux disease (GERD). Although there is some overlap between esophageal motor disorders associated with dysphagia and the defects and esophageal motor function that would predispose the patient to more severe GERD, this review is organized to differentiate the distinct pathophysiologic components of the two disease groups. The section on dysphagia provides a description of disorders associated with esophagogastric junction (EGJ) outflow obstruction and disorders of contractility associated with premature spastic contractions, hypercontractility, and impaired bolus clearance. By contrast, the section on GERD focuses on a description of an incompetent EGJ and antireflux barrier. A section on impaired bolus transit is also included to highlight the important aspect of impaired clearance in the pathogenesis of GERD.

DYSPHAGIA

Dysphagia will typically result secondary to either an obstruction to flow or an inability to adequately propel the bolus in the antegrade direction into the stomach. Thus, an atlas focused on describing disorders associated with the symptom of dysphagia should highlight examples of EGJ outflow obstruction and abnormalities of contraction associated with impaired antegrade flow.

EGJ Obstruction

The measurement of the pressure changes through the EGJ during swallowing is much more complex than previously understood. The EGJ is a complex anatomic zone that maintains a closed state at baseline via a delicate interplay between neurogenic, myogenic, and mechanical properties. During swallowing, the lower esophageal sphincter (LES) normally relaxes to allow bolus transit through the EGJ. However, other factors also impede flow by resisting opening during bolus transit. The hiatal canal is usually the narrowest diameter through the EGJ[3] and thus, this will be the primary determinant of flow rate through the

EGJ. In addition, there are other mechanical properties of the esophageal wall that will also resist opening secondary to elastic properties of the EGJ. Therefore, the pressure signal through the EGJ during swallowing can be altered by dysfunction of LES relaxation and a reduced opening diameter related to a mechanical obstruction (stricture, eosinophilic esophagitis, tumor, LES hypertrophy)[4] or abnormal anatomy (hiatus hernia).[5]

The two measurements that are important in defining EGJ outflow obstruction are the integrated relaxation pressure (IRP) and the intrabolus pressurization pattern.[6,7] The IRP is a complex metric, as it involves accurately localizing the margins of the EGJ, demarcating the time window following deglutitive upper sphincter relaxation within which to anticipate EGJ relaxation to occur, applying an e-sleeve measurement (axial EGJ

domain) within that 10-second time box (**Fig. 2**). The IRP is presented as the mean value of the 4 seconds during which the e-sleeve value was least. Patients that exhibit an abnormal IRP and/or an elevated intrabolus pressurization have evidence of EGJ outflow obstruction; however, the specific cause cannot be discriminated purely by manometric evaluation of the EGJ alone. Thus the distinction of achalasia from other disorders associated with EGJ outflow obstruction will require further evaluation of the pathognomonic contractile and pressure patterns in addition to a detailed description of the EGJ anatomy (**Fig. 3**).

Achalasia

Achalasia is defined by an increased IRP and absent peristalsis, and can be further subtyped into 3 specific groups based on the characteristics that are associated with absent peristalsis. Type I

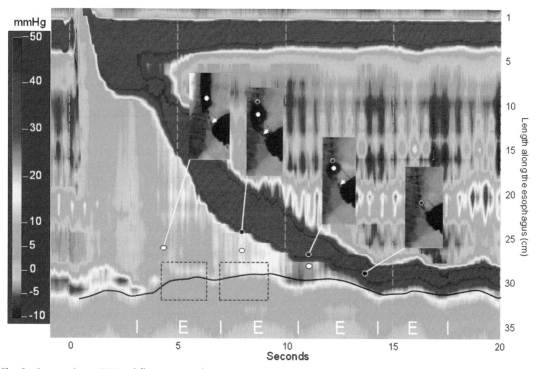

Fig. 2. Concomitant EPT and fluoroscopy during esophageal emptying, illustrating the transition from peristaltic transport to ampullary emptying. The fluoroscopic images in the windows are synchronized with the EPT plot. The white and blue dots indicate areas of intrabolus pressure and the onset of luminal closure, respectively. The second image (at about time 8 seconds) is near the contractile deceleration point (CDP), evident by both the transition of the fluoroscopic image to ampullary conformation and slowing of the luminal closure front. The dashed rectangles within the deglutitive relaxation window indicate the time fragments used to compute the integrated relaxation pressure (IRP). The distal border of the esophagogastric junction (EGJ) is indicated by a black line on EPT and by white arrows on barium swallow. Note that the pressure signal through the two boxes that demarcate the IRP measurement are a manifestation of the compartmentalized intrabolus pressure between the EGJ and the contractile wavefront. Thus, this measurement provides a measure of the pressure gradient across the EGJ and it therefore is not a one-dimensional measure of lower esophageal sphincter (LES) relaxation.

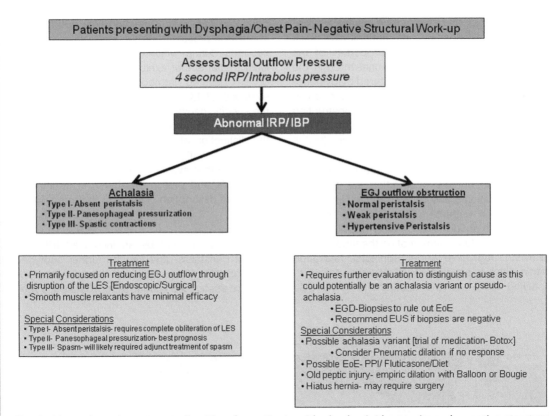

Fig. 3. Diagnosis and treatment algorithm for patients with dysphagia/chest pain and negative structural workup. EPT study allows an assessment of distal outflow pressure. An abnormal integrated relaxation pressure (IRP) and/or abnormal intrabolus pressure (IBP) defines that an esophagogastric junction (EGJ) outflow obstruction is present and that further diagnosis requires an analysis of contractile activity. In conjunction with absent peristalsis, achalasia is diagnosed. The treatment will then focus on reducing EGJ outflow obstruction. When esophageal peristalsis is preserved (normal, weak, or hypertensive), the pattern is distinguished from achalasia and is defined as EGJ outflow obstruction. Further evaluations are then required to ascertain the cause of obstruction. EGD, esophagogastroduodenoscopy; EoE, eosinophilic esophagitis; EUS, endoscopic ultrasonography; LES, lower esophageal sphincter; PPI, proton-pump inhibitors.

achalasia is associated with 100% failed peristalsis and no evidence of contractile activity or pressurization greater than 30 mm Hg (**Fig. 4**A). Type II achalasia is also associated with no normal peristalsis and no significant contractile activity, but is distinguished from type I based on the presence of pan-esophageal pressurization greater than 30 mm Hg (see **Fig. 4**B). Type III achalasia manifests absent peristalsis in the context of preserved fragments of contraction or premature spastic contractions greater than or equal to 20% of the swallow's studied space (see **Fig. 4**C). The clinical relevance of this classification subtype has been assessed in 3 studies.[8–10] These studies support that type II has the best prognosis, whereas type I is worse than type II but much better than type III. Type III patients will still manifest spastic contractions within the body of the esophagus, and will require treatment above the EGJ that is focused on reducing the spastic contractions.

EGJ outflow obstruction

EGJ outflow obstruction is defined by an abnormal IRP and/or elevated intrabolus pressure in the context of some instances of intact peristalsis or weak peristalsis, with small breaks such that the criteria for achalasia are not met.[4] This condition may be related to a mechanical obstruction secondary to a stricture (**Fig. 5**A), or an anatomic defect such as a hernia (see **Fig. 5**B). In addition, this pattern can be seen in patients with postsurgical complications at the EGJ (fundoplication) or the proximal stomach (lap band).

Spastic Disorders

The major pathologic features of spastic disorders of the esophagus are premature contractions defined by reduced latency and rapid contractions with normal latency. The 3 measurements important in defining spastic disorders are noted in

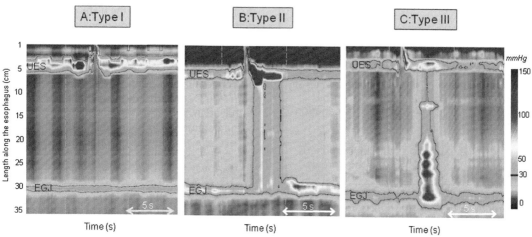

Fig. 4. Achalasia subtypes. All 3 subtypes are characterized by impaired EGJ relaxation (IRP >15 mm Hg) and absent contractile activity. In type I (*A*) there is negligible pressurization in the esophageal body, evident by the absence of any area circumscribed by the 30-mm Hg isobaric contour (*black line*). In type II (*B*) panesophageal pressurization occurs, evident by the banding pattern of the 30-mm Hg isobaric contour spanning from the upper esophageal sphincter (UES) to the esophagogastric junction (EGJ). This depiction represents elevated intrabolus pressure, and is associated with contraction of the longitudinal muscle on the muscularis propria. Type III achalasia (*C*) is characterized by spastic contractions with or without periods of compartmentalized pressurization.

Table 1 and are described in **Figs. 6** and **7**. Before the appropriate measurements can be made, two important landmarks must be established: onset of swallowing and the contractile deceleration point (CDP).[11] Once these landmarks are established, measurements of contractile front velocity and distal latency can be made. The latency interval is a measurement that defines the zone of normal deglutitive inhibition through the smooth-muscle esophagus.[12] Contractions where the CDP occurs within 4.5 seconds of the initiation of the swallow defined by the upper esophageal sphincter are likely associated with impaired inhibition in the smooth-muscle esophagus and bolus entrapment

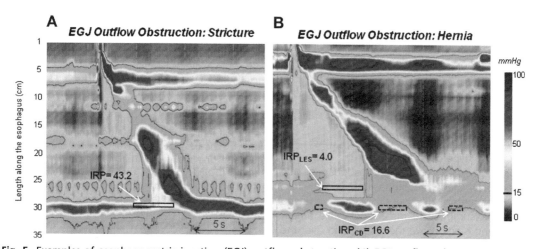

Fig. 5. Examples of esophagogastric junction (EGJ) outflow obstruction. (*A*) EGJ outflow obstruction occurs in a context of stricture. It is characterized by an elevated IRP and a distal compartmentalization. (*B*) EGJ outflow obstruction occurs in a context of hiatal hernia. The hernia is evidenced on Clouse plots by the separation between the lower esophageal sphincter (LES) and the crural diaphragm (CD). In this case, IRP is restricted to the LES (*black box*, IRP$_{LES}$) and CD (*black dashed boxes*, IRP$_{CD}$) separately. The CD component of the basal EGJ pressure profile is quite pronounced. A compartmentalized pressurization occurred between the contractile wave and the CD, reflecting the greater resistance through the CD evidenced by elevated IRP$_{CD}$ (16.6 mm Hg).

Table 1
Important measures in assessing contractile propagation

CDP (time, position) *Contractile Deceleration Point*	The inflection point along the 30-mm Hg isobaric contour where propagation velocity slows, demarcating the tubular esophagus from the phrenic ampulla
CFV (cm/s) *Contractile Front Velocity*	Slope of the tangent approximating the 30-mm Hg isobaric contour between proximal trough and the CDP
DL (s) *Distal Latency*	Interval between upper esophageal sphincter relaxation and the CDP

(see **Fig. 7**).[13] Rapid contractions are defined by contractile velocity greater than 9 cm/s; however, this particular parameter must be evaluated in the context of latency.[11] Swallows with rapid contraction and normal latency do not exhibit impaired inhibition in the smooth-muscle esophagus, and thus are different from the classic spastic disorders that are associated with the corkscrew esophagus or rosary-bead esophagus on fluoroscopy. The different phenotypes of spastic disorders are illustrated in **Fig. 8**.[14] The clinical implications of rapid contractions with normal latency are unclear; however, rapid contractions associated with reduced distal latency comprise a distinct pathophysiologic entity never encountered in asymptomatic control populations.

Hypercontractile Disorders

The classic hypercontractile disorder was originally described as "nutcracker" esophagus, due to the high peristaltic amplitudes noted on conventional manometry.[15] Current definitions are based on the measurement of mean contractile amplitudes 3 and 8 cm above the LES,[16] and over the years some experts have called for a more stringent definition to better define this pathophysiologic clinical entity.[17] With this call to better define hypercontractile disorders, the EPT classification of hypertensive contractile disorders has also sought to separate clinically significant phenotypes of hypercontractility. A new metric to

define hypercontractility, the distal contractile integral (DCI), was devised to summarize the vigor of the distal esophageal contraction measured for the segment spanning from the proximal (P) to distal (D) pressure troughs (**Fig. 9**). The DCI can be conceptualized as the volume of the pressure from P to D, thereby being sensitive to the length of that span, as well as the amplitude and duration of the contraction at each locus along the way.[17] To exclude the effects of intrabolus pressure in the DCI computation, the first 20 mm Hg is ignored.[18,19] Consequently, if a swallow was not associated with any recorded pressure greater than 20 mm Hg in the P to D span, the DCI for that swallow would be zero. However, keep in mind that the DCI was devised primarily to identify swallows of excessive contractile vigor, making the upper rather than the lower limit of normal the more relevant limit. The upper limit of normal defined by the 95th percentile in a normal population is 5000 mm Hg-s-cm, whereas when defined

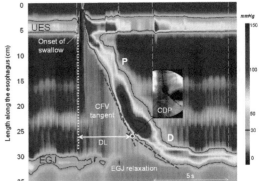

Fig. 6. A normal swallow in a Clouse plot. Before and after the swallow, two high-pressure zones are visualized: the upper esophageal sphincter (UES) and the esophagogastric junction (EGJ). The highlighted black line is the 30-mm Hg isobaric contour circumscribing areas on the plot with intraluminal pressure greater than 30 mm Hg. The peristaltic esophageal contraction is characterized by two troughs, one proximal (P) and one distal (D). The contractile deceleration point (CDP) represents the inflexion point in the contractile front propagation. It is localized on Clouse plots by fitting two tangential lines to the initial and terminal portions of the 30-mm Hg isobaric contours and noting intersection of the lines (*white dot*). On fluoroscopic image it corresponds to the transition to ampullary conformation and slowing of the luminal closure front. The contractile front velocity (CFV) corresponds to the slope of the tangent line to the initial portion of the contraction (between P and the CDP). The distal latency (DL) is measured from the onset of swallow (dashed vertical line) to the CDP.

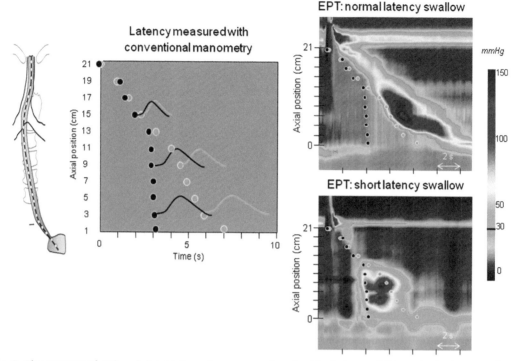

Fig. 7. The concept of reduced distal latency in spasm as described by Behar and Biancani. The latency of propagation for normal controls (*black circles*) and a patient with spasm (*orange circles*) adapted from Behar and Biancani (*left panel*). The latency interval was measured using conventional manometry, as the time from onset of contraction at sensor 21 to onset of contraction at sensor 1. The latency interval was determined to be a marker of the inhibitory ganglionic integrity, suggesting that patients with spasm had evidence of reduced latency and premature contraction. In the right panels, the latency interval plots from the conventional manometry study are superimposed on esophageal pressure topography (EPT) tracings of a swallow with normal latency (*top*) and short latency (*bottom*). In each case, the time and sensor position scales are adjusted to approximate those of the conventional manometry tracing. (*Data from (Left panel)*: Behar J, Biancani P. Pathogenesis of simultaneous esophageal contractions in patients with motility disorders. Gastroenterology 1993;105(1):111–8; and *Courtesy of* The Northwestern University HRM Database; with permission.)

by the value never encountered in a normal population it is 8000 mm Hg-s-cm.[19,20]

Weak and Failed Peristalsis

The importance of weak and failed peristalsis in the pathogenesis of dysphagia is unclear, therefore these motor disorders are more fully discussed in the section on GERD. However, two specific disorders do deserve special mention. Absent peristalsis is characterized by failed peristalsis with 100% of swallows. This disorder is uniformly associated with poor bolus transit, and this motor pattern is associated with type I achalasia (see **Fig. 4**A) and the scleroderma pattern if the patient has a hypotensive LES. Absent peristalsis can occasionally be found in the context of a normal LES pressure and intact deglutitive EGJ relaxation. These patients will also be predisposed to poor esophageal clearance and will therefore be susceptible to more severe GERD,

and possibly postfundoplication dysphagia.[21] A distinct form of weak peristalsis associated with a defect in the transition zone or the proximal trough can be associated with dysphagia and poor proximal bolus clearance.[2,22,23] These patients may be susceptible to pill esophagitis and proximal regurgitation (see the section on impaired esophageal clearance).

GASTROESOPHAGEAL REFLUX

The primary determinants of GERD severity are a dysfunctional antireflux barrier and impaired esophageal clearance. The antireflux barrier prevents reflux of gastric contents into the esophagus while peristalsis helps to clear the refluxate to reduce exposure to the noxious components of the gastric juice. The primary mechanisms of reflux have focused on 3 dominant mechanisms: (1) transient LES relaxations (tLESRs), without anatomic

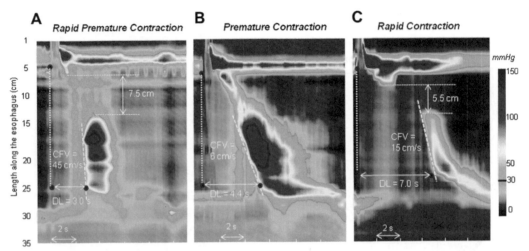

Fig. 8. Examples of premature and rapid esophageal contractions. Premature contraction is defined by a distal latency (DL, measured from onset of swallow to the contractile deceleration point) of less than 4.5 seconds. Rapid contraction is defined by a contractile front velocity (CFV, measured from the proximal trough to the CDP) of greater than 9 cm/s. The contraction on (*A*) is rapid and premature, and this represents a manometric description of the "corkscrew" or "rosary bead" esophagus. Note that this contraction is associated with a large proximal defect. The contraction on (*B*) is premature with a normal CFV, and occurred in a context of an abnormal esophagogastric junction (EGJ) relaxation. This pattern is extremely rare and is typically associated with evidence of obstruction at the EGJ. The contraction on (*C*) is rapid with a normal DL, and is associated with a large proximal defect. This pattern is found in asymptomatic controls and is associated with poor bolus transit related to the defect in the contractile wavefront.

abnormality, (2) LES hypotension, again without anatomic abnormality, or (3) anatomic distortion of the EGJ inclusive of (but not limited to) hiatus hernia. Once the gastroesophageal refluxate enters the esophagus, peristalsis functions to clear the esophagus of the refluxate. Defects in the integrity of the peristaltic wave will lead to impaired bolus transit and prolonged esophageal

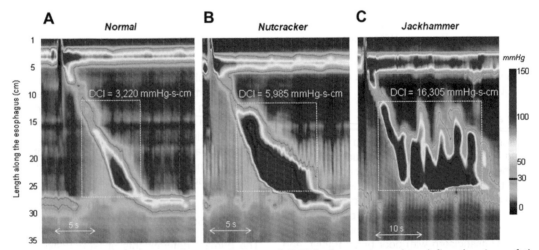

Fig. 9. Hypertensive peristalsis. Distal contractile integral (DCI) is the metric used to define the vigor of the contraction. It is the product of the amplitude × duration × length of the contraction between the proximal and the distal trough. The contraction exhibited in (*A*) is normal. A hypertensive contraction defined by a DCI greater than 5000 mm Hg-s-cm is presented in (*B*). This contraction occurs in a context of normal propagation and normal esophagogastric junction (EGJ) relaxation. Nutcracker esophagus is defined by a mean DCI of 10 swallows greater than 5000 mm Hg-s-cm in a context of normal propagation and normal EGJ relaxation. (*C*) Illustrates an extreme phenotype of hypertensive contraction characterized by a DCI greater than 8000 mm Hg-s-cm and repetitive prolonged contractions evoking the action of the jackhammer. This extreme phenotype is named jackhammer contraction, and is never found in asymptomatic controls.

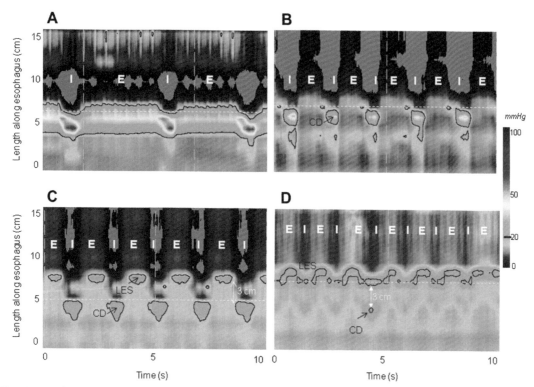

Fig. 10. Esophagogastric junction (EGJ) morphology characterized in Clouse plots. The two main EGJ components are lower esophageal sphincter (LES) and crural diaphragm (CD), which cannot be independently quantified when superimposed, classified as type I EGJ (*A*). The respiratory inversion point (RIP), shown by the horizontal dashed line, lies at the proximal margin of the EGJ. During the expiration (E) EGJ pressure increases, whereas it decreases during inspiration (I). In the case of hypotensive EGJ only the diaphragmatic component is identified (*B*). (*C*) and (*D*) correspond to type III EGJ defined as LES-CD separation greater than 2 cm. A type III EGJ is the manometric criterion for hiatal hernia. The RIP is within the EGJ at the proximal margin of the CD. Two subtypes were discernible, IIIa (*C*) and IIIb (*D*), with the distinction being that the RIP was proximal to the CD with IIIa and proximal to the LES in IIIb.

acid exposure. This exposure is a critical component of the pathogenesis of GERD, and prolonged exposure times are associated with more severe GERD.

Antireflux Barrier

Disruption of the antireflux barrier can be related to a hypotensive LES (<10 mm Hg),[24] an abnormal gastroesophageal flap valve,[25] radial disruption of the crural canal,[26] and hiatus hernia. These defects are not mutually exclusive, and the defects are cumulative in terms of their effect on disrupting the antireflux barrier. HRM and EPT allow one to accurately assess the intrinsic LES and the crural component contribution to the EGJ high-pressure zone (**Fig. 10**). The crural component can be assessed by measuring the inspiratory augmentation during baseline recordings, and recent data suggest that this measurement may be a predictor of GERD.[27]

In addition, the separation between the intrinsic LES and crural diaphragm can be measured simultaneously during HRM studies to document the presence of hiatus hernia.[28] In addition, localization of the respiratory inversion point can provide some insight into the level of crural disruption (see **Fig. 10**).

Impaired Esophageal Clearance

Patients with weak or failed peristalsis will have an impaired ability to clear the refluxate after gastroesophageal reflux occurs. The degree of impairment is likely a function of the number of failed peristaltic events, and whether the peristaltic contraction is intact or associated with breaks in the peristaltic wavefront (**Fig. 11**). Patients with absent peristalsis have the most severe impairment in esophageal clearance, and thus are likely to have the most severe GERD. If this is associated with a hypotensive LES, a diagnosis of scleroderma

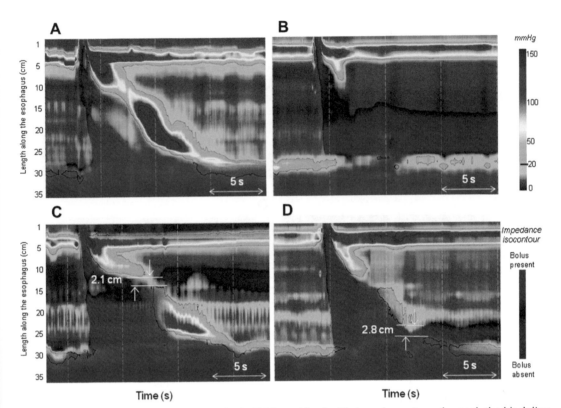

Fig. 11. Varying degrees of peristaltic integrity in HRM combined with impedance. In each panel, the black line represents the 20-mm Hg isobaric contour (IBC). Impedance data are displayed by overlaid pink colorization, with the pink shading indicating areas on the topography plots with retained bolus. The swallow in (*A*) is intact (no disruption in the 20-mm Hg IBC) and is associated with complete bolus transit. (*B*) Illustrates a failed swallow (absence of 20-mm Hg integrity in the distal two-thirds of the esophagus) associated with bolus retention in the esophagus. Swallows with small break in the 20-mm Hg IBC are illustrated in (*C*) and (*D*). The transition zone break is responsible for bolus escape in (*C*). In (*D*) the distal break is associated with bolus retention in the distal esophagus, and corresponds to what has been previously defined as ineffective esophageal motility.

must be considered; however, this pattern is not pathognomonic for this disease and can be seen in the context of severe GERD (**Fig. 12**). Another esophageal motor defect associated with GERD is ineffective esophageal motility. Classically this entity was defined as a peristaltic amplitude less than 30 mm Hg in the conventional recording sites located in the distal esophagus 3 and 8 cm above the LES.[29] In HRM, this definition has changed by leveraging the spatial resolution of HRM to measure the actual defect lengths in the contractile wavefronts. Recent work by Roman and colleagues[30] has defined that defects greater than 5 cm are uniformly associated with impaired bolus transit. Although confirmatory studies are needed, it is likely reasonable to equate distal defects in the contractile wavefront with swallows associated with ineffective esophageal motility.

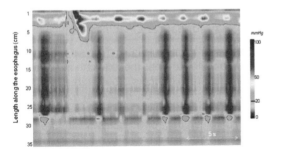

Fig. 12. Scleroderma. The typical pattern is characterized by hypotensive lower esophageal sphincter pressure and absence of contraction in the distal two-thirds of the esophagus.

REFERENCES

1. Clouse RE, Staiano A. Topography of the esophageal peristaltic pressure wave. Am J Physiol 1991; 261(4 Pt 1):G677–84.
2. Fox M, Hebbard G, Janiak P, et al. High-resolution manometry predicts the success of oesophageal bolus transport and identifies clinically important

abnormalities not detected by conventional manometry. Neurogastroenterol Motil 2004;16(5):533–42.

3. Pandolfino JE, Shi G, Curry J, et al. Esophagogastric junction distensibility: a factor contributing to sphincter incompetence. Am J Physiol Gastrointest Liver Physiol 2002;282(6):G1052–8.

4. Scherer JR, Kwiatek MA, Soper NJ, et al. Functional esophagogastric junction obstruction with intact peristalsis: a heterogeneous syndrome sometimes akin to achalasia. J Gastrointest Surg 2009;13(12):2219–25.

5. Pandolfino JE, Kwiatek MA, Ho K, et al. Unique features of esophagogastric junction pressure topography in hiatus hernia patients with dysphagia. Surgery 2010;147(1):57–64.

6. Pandolfino JE, Ghosh SK, Zhang Q, et al. Quantifying EGJ morphology and relaxation with high-resolution manometry: a study of 75 asymptomatic volunteers. Am J Physiol Gastrointest Liver Physiol 2006;290(5):G1033–40.

7. Ghosh SK, Pandolfino JE, Rice J, et al. Impaired deglutitive EGJ relaxation in clinical esophageal manometry: a quantitative analysis of 400 patients and 75 controls. Am J Physiol Gastrointest Liver Physiol 2007;293(4):G878–85.

8. Pandolfino JE, Kwiatek MA, Nealis T, et al. Achalasia: a new clinically relevant classification by high-resolution manometry. Gastroenterology 2008;135(5):1526–33.

9. Salvador R, Costantini M, Zaninotto G, et al. The preoperative manometric pattern predicts the outcome of surgical treatment for esophageal achalasia. J Gastrointest Surg 2010;14(11):1635–45.

10. Pratap N, Reddy DN. Can achalasia subtyping by high-resolution manometry predict the therapeutic outcome of pneumatic balloon dilatation?: author's reply. J Neurogastroenterol Motil 2011;17(2):205.

11. Pandolfino JE, Leslie E, Luger D, et al. The contractile deceleration point: an important physiologic landmark on oesophageal pressure topography. Neurogastroenterol Motil 2010;22(4):395–400, e90.

12. Behar J, Biancani P. Pathogenesis of simultaneous esophageal contractions in patients with motility disorders. Gastroenterology 1993;105(1):111–8.

13. Roman S, Lin Z, Pandolfino JE, et al. Distal contraction latency: a measure of propagation velocity optimized for esophageal pressure topography studies. Am J Gastroenterol 2011;106(3):443–51.

14. Pandolfino JE, Roman S, Carlson D, et al. Distal esophageal spasm in high-resolution esophageal pressure topography: defining clinical phenotypes. Gastroenterology 2011;141(2):469–75.

15. Benjamin SB, Gerhardt DC, Castell DO. High amplitude, peristaltic esophageal contractions associated with chest pain and/or dysphagia. Gastroenterology 1979;77(3):478–83.

16. Spechler SJ, Castell DO. Classification of oesophageal motility abnormalities. Gut 2001;49(1):145–51.

17. Agrawal A, Hila A, Tutuian R, et al. Clinical relevance of the nutcracker esophagus: suggested revision of criteria for diagnosis. J Clin Gastroenterol 2006;40(6):504–9.

18. Ghosh SK, Pandolfino JE, Zhang Q, et al. Quantifying esophageal peristalsis with high-resolution manometry: a study of 75 asymptomatic volunteers. Am J Physiol Gastrointest Liver Physiol 2006;290(5):G988–97.

19. Pandolfino JE, Fox MR, Bredenoord AJ, et al. High-resolution manometry in clinical practice: utilizing pressure topography to classify oesophageal motility abnormalities. Neurogastroenterol Motil 2009;21(8):796–806.

20. Roman S, Lin Z, Kwiatek MA, et al. Jackhammer esophagus: a symptomatic phenotype of hypertensive contraction in high resolution esophageal pressure topography (EPT). Gastroenterology 2011;140(5 Suppl 1):S-231.

21. Fibbe C, Layer P, Keller J, et al. Esophageal motility in reflux disease before and after fundoplication: a prospective, randomized, clinical, and manometric study. Gastroenterology 2001;121(1):5–14.

22. Ghosh SK, Pandolfino JE, Kwiatek MA, et al. Oesophageal peristaltic transition zone defects: real but few and far between. Neurogastroenterol Motil 2008;20(12):1283–90.

23. Pohl D, Ribolsi M, Savarino E, et al. Characteristics of the esophageal low-pressure zone in healthy volunteers and patients with esophageal symptoms: assessment by high-resolution manometry. Am J Gastroenterol 2008;103(10):2544–9.

24. Sloan S, Rademaker AW, Kahrilas PJ. Determinants of gastroesophageal junction incompetence: hiatal hernia, lower esophageal sphincter, or both? Ann Intern Med 1992;117(12):977–82.

25. Hill LD, Kozarek RA, Kraemer SJ, et al. The gastroesophageal flap valve: in vitro and in vivo observations. Gastrointest Endosc 1996;44(5):541–7.

26. Pandolfino JE, Shi G, Trueworthy B, et al. Esophagogastric junction opening during relaxation distinguishes nonhernia reflux patients, hernia patients, and normal subjects. Gastroenterology 2003;125(4):1018–24.

27. Pandolfino JE, Kim H, Ghosh SK, et al. High-resolution manometry of the EGJ: an analysis of crural diaphragm function in GERD. Am J Gastroenterol 2007;102(5):1056–63.

28. Pandolfino JE, El-Serag HB, Zhang Q, et al. Obesity: a challenge to esophagogastric junction integrity. Gastroenterology 2006;130(3):639–49.

29. Leite LP, Johnston BT, Barrett J, et al. Ineffective esophageal motility (IEM): the primary finding in patients with nonspecific esophageal motility disorder. Dig Dis Sci 1997;42(9):1859–65.

30. Roman S, Lin Z, Kwiatek MA, et al. Weak peristalsis in esophageal pressure topography: classification and association with Dysphagia. Am J Gastroenterol 2011;106(2):349–56.

Evaluation and Treatment of Laryngopharyngeal Reflux Symptoms

Yong S. Kwon, MD[a], Brant K. Oelschlager, MD[b],*,
Albert L. Merati, MD[c]

KEYWORDS

- Gastrointestinal reflux disease • Laryngopharyngeal reflux
- Laryngospasm • Extraesophageal symptoms

Gastroesophageal reflux disease (GERD) is a well-defined disease characterized by symptoms or complications caused by an abnormal amount of gastroesophageal reflux (GER), which is a retrograde movement of gastric contents into the esophagus. An estimated 25 to 75 million people in the United States are affected by GERD, and 13% of Americans use medications at least twice weekly.[1] Laryngopharyngeal reflux (LPR) is considered a subset of GERD and its own identity, because the main symptomatic region involves the laryngopharynx. Although the hallmark symptoms of GERD include heartburn and regurgitation, symptoms of LPR often include cough, throat discomfort, and hoarseness, which are also termed *extraesophageal symptoms*. In some patients with LPR, the extraesophageal symptoms occur in conjunction with classic symptoms, whereas in others the respiratory symptoms are the only manifestations of GER.

Increased interest has been shown in LPR in the past 10 to 15 years. LPR has become one of the more frequently diagnosed conditions in otolaryngology.[2] It has been reported that up to 10% of otolaryngologic clinic patients overall and approximately 50% of patients with voice complaints have been diagnosed with LPR.[3] LPR has been linked to several disorders, including chronic laryngitis, chronic dysphonia, chronic cough, asthma, laryngotracheal stenosis, vocal cord lesions, and laryngospasm. Pathophysiology of LPR is likely multifactorial. Numerous studies have been undertaken to clarify the pathophysiology of LPR, and these have shown that both direct refluxate contact of the laryngopharynx and indirect reflexive laryngospasm likely account for symptoms of LPR. Accurate diagnosis of LPR has been elusive, but implementation of direct reflux monitoring using pH probe and impedance studies in addition to laryngoscopies have proven useful. This article describes other diagnostic modalities on the horizon that may offer improved diagnostic accuracy. The treatment of LPR has been similar to that of GERD. Lifestyle modifications and medical and surgical treatment have had mixed results.

Although evaluation and treatment of LPR has been challenging, promising progress has been made in delineating the complex pathophysiology and realizing the wide array of clinical manifestations. In addition, advancements have been made in developing new diagnostic tools and understanding how to treat patients with LPR.

[a] Department of Surgery, Center for Videoendoscopic Surgery, University of Washington, Seattle, WA, USA
[b] Department of Surgery, Center for Videoendoscopic Surgery, Center for Esophageal and Gastric Surgery, University of Washington, 1959 NE Pacific Street, Box 356410, Seattle, WA 98195, USA
[c] Department of Otolaryngology, University of Washington, 1959 NE Pacific Street, Box 356161, Seattle, WA 98195, USA
* Corresponding author.
E-mail address: brant@uw.edu

Thorac Surg Clin 21 (2011) 477–487
doi:10.1016/j.thorsurg.2011.08.001
1547-4127/11/$ – see front matter © 2011 Published by Elsevier Inc

PATHOPHYSIOLOGY
Physiology

The origin of reflux events that occur with GERD is well delineated. The lower esophageal sphincter (LES) has the most critical role in preventing gastric refluxate from entering the esophagus. The LES is a physiologic entity characterized by high-pressure zone just cephalad to the gastro-esophageal junction. This high-pressure zone is reinforced by intrinsic musculature of the distal esophagus, the sling fibers of the cardia, and the diaphragm. A competent LES has a tonic resting pressure that is greater than the gastric pressure. This tonic contraction of the LES results in closure that prevents the reflux. Relaxation of the LES occurs during swallowing, belching, and vomiting.

GER can occur when the sphincter with normal tonic pressure undergoes transient spontaneous relaxation. This transient relaxation is present even in a normal healthy population. GER can also occur when the integrity of the high-pressure zone is compromised to a degree at which it is unable to prevent gastric refluxate from entering the esophagus. A pathologic example of this scenario includes a large hiatal hernia in which the relationship between the LES and the diaphragmatic crura is displaced. A physiologic example of this scenario includes stress reflux elicited by heavy lifting, straining, and coughing during which intraabdominal pressure exceeds the LES pressure. Although some degree of reflux is present in most individuals, GERD is diagnosed when the presentation and evaluation of characteristics are consistent with an abnormal amount of GER.

LPR represents extension of GER into the larynx, pharynx, and upper aerodigestive tract. Aside from the LES, three other barriers prevent reflux to this proximal extent: the upper esophageal sphincter (UES), intrinsic esophageal acid clearance, and the esophageal epithelial resistance.[3] Although different reflex mechanisms, such as laryngopharyngeal chemoreflex and vagally mediated reflexes, have been known to cause symptoms of LPR, dysfunction within these three components may also contribute to manifestations of LPR.

The upper esophageal sphincter
The UES is a functional entity of the distal pharynx and the proximal esophagus that maintains a closed state via tonic contraction of the cricopharyngeus. During specific demands such as belching and swallowing, the UES relaxes. The UES tonic pressure is increased in response to laryngeal stimulation, acidification of the distal esophagus, and distension of the lower esophagus.[4,5]

Smoking is also known to lower the UES pressure and inhibit contractile reflexes that would normally aid in airway protection.

Intrinsic esophageal acid clearance mechanism
The esophagus has chemical and mechanical defenses against refluxate other than the UES and the LES. Tonic production of salivary bicarbonate occurs, which works to protect its surface from acidic refluxate by neutralization. Another intrinsic clearance mechanism involves esophageal peristalsis, which mechanically clears the esophagus of its contents. Ineffective peristalsis, therefore, can result in greater contact time between the gastric refluxate and the esophageal mucosa, thus increasing the damage from any given amount of refluxed acid and other gastric components.

Esophageal epithelial resistance
Properties of the esophageal epithelium serve to protect it from the gastric refluxate. The epithelium is covered by a mucus layer and an aqueous layer with a high bicarbonate content.[4] The mucus layer protects by acting as a physical barriers to offending agents such as pepsin. The concentrated bicarbonate layer buffers against the acidic contents of the gastric refluxate. However, the resistance property of the esophageal epithelium is more robust than that of the respiratory epithelium. Laryngeal epithelium does not possess the ability to actively produce bicarbonate, rendering itself vulnerable in the event of acidic proximal GER.

Mechanism

Several mechanisms have been proposed through which symptoms of LPR are manifested, but these generally fall into the category of direct contact of refluxate or reflex responses to GER.

Direct epithelial contact
The most likely cause of LPR symptoms is for injury to occur secondary to retrograde flow of gastric contents making direct contact with the laryngeal and pharyngeal epithelium. A recent experiment designed to study the effects of acidic reflux on the vocal fold showed that transepithelial resistance was irreversibly and substantially reduced when porcine vocal folds were exposed to physiologically relevant acidic pepsin and acid alone.[6] This direct contact may also give rise to mucosal ulceration, generalized inflammatory response, and necrosis.[3] The squamous respiratory epithelium of the posterior larynx that normally functions to clear mucus may also be damaged as a result of the gastric refluxate. Resultant injury to

the squamous epithelium leads to stasis of the mucus, which can lead to postnasal drip and increased throat clearing.[7] When compared with the esophageal mucosa, the upper respiratory epithelium is significantly more vulnerable secondary to lack of defenses, and even short bursts of direct contact with gastric refluxate can lead to vocal cord edema, contact ulcers, and granulomas.

The laryngopharyngeal damage may be caused partly by acid, but it likely involves other components. One factor that has been shown to play a role in pathogenesis of LPR is pepsin. Pepsin is a proteolytic enzyme that takes its active form from pepsinogen secreted by the gastric chief cells. Pepsinogen is cleaved by hydrochloric acid in the stomach. Pepsin is maximally active at a pH of 2 but it can cause tissue damage at a pH up to 6.5.[8] Johnston and colleagues[9] showed that pepsin is found in human laryngeal epithelium gathered from patients with reflux-attributed laryngeal disease. This expression of pepsin in the laryngeal epithelium was absent in patients without symptoms. Pepsin has been hypothesized to cause cellular damage through different mechanisms. First, experiments have shown that certain mucosa-protective proteins, including carbonic anhydrase III, are expressed in a decreased amount in patients with LPR compared with normal subjects. In the same patient group, pepsin was present in high concentrations. This finding led some to believe that pepsin, when activated in the laryngopharynx, can cause dysfunction of the mucosa-protective protein response.[10] Second, pepsin can disrupt cellular integrity through its proteolytic activity, which can digest the molecules that maintain cohesions between cells. Whether activated by short bursts of an acidic environment created from reflux, or by the acidic intracellular compartments encountered after receptor-mediated endocytosis, pepsin has been postulated to be one of the main destructive players with its proteolytic capacity. In addition, studies have shown pepsin-inducing expression of proinflammatory cytokines and receptors, including those involved in the esophageal epithelial inflammation that contributes to the pathophysiology of reflux esophagitis.[11] Although the details of pepsin's role in pathophysiology of LPR is still being investigated, the current body of study indicates that pepsin may be one of the main mediators of LPR.

Laryngeal and pharyngeal reflexes

Laryngospasm is a sudden forceful apposition of the vocal cords and can occur as result of a noxious stimuli.[12] Symptoms of LPR may be induced by laryngospasm caused by two different potential reflex loops.[13] The proposed reflexive mechanism is not necessarily from the epithelial injuries caused by direct refluxate contact.

The first reflexive mechanism that can result in laryngospasm is the laryngeal chemoreflex. The reflex pathway consists of an afferent limb carried by the stimulated superior laryngeal nerve (SLN) and an efferent limb carried by the recurrent laryngeal nerve (RLN).[14] This reflex arc is stimulated by refluxed material, which results in vocal cord adduction and laryngospasm.[15] The authors who first described this reflex arc showed that electrical stimulation of the SLN produced repetitive, excitatory discharges of the RLN, which led to adduction of the vocal cords through stimulation of the thyroarytenoid and lateral cricoarytenoid muscles.[14]

The second reflexive mechanism that can result in LPR symptoms is the vagally mediated reflex elicited by stimulation of the distal esophagus. Animal studies have shown that sensory stimulation of the distal esophagus in the absence of any laryngeal stimulation can cause laryngospasm via an afferent limb of the vagus nerve. This vagally mediated reflex has also been associated with other entities, such as sudden infant death syndrome.[13]

As a result of these reflex mechanisms alone, patients may experience symptoms of LPR. When diagnosing and treating LPR, providers must be mindful that symptoms of laryngospasm could be caused by these reflex mechanisms rather than a direct insult to the larynx and pharynx from gastroesophageal refluxate.

Spectrum of Disease

LPR as an entity can manifest in a wide variety of symptoms. Its clinical sequelae can range from benign transient voice changes to advanced laryngeal cancers. Careful evaluations of patient histories are important in diagnosing LPR.[2] Patients may present with one or several of a wide array of symptoms, including hoarseness, globus sensation, throat clearing, postnasal drip sensation, dysphagia, chronic cough, choking sensation, and heartburn. LPR should be suspected when clinical history and initial findings are suggestive. One of the more frequent presenting symptoms of LPR is hoarseness.[16] Hoarseness can be caused by inflammatory, neoplastic, neurologic, or phonotraumatic disorders, to name several broad categories. The characteristics of hoarseness can be used to help narrow down the origin. With LPR, the hoarseness often fluctuates and is sometimes associated with throat discomfort; it is often accompanied by cough and throat clearing. On laryngeal examination, vocal fold edema, erythema, and pseudosulcus are useful findings.[17] Granulomata, when present, are also highly suggestive of LPR.[18] Laryngoscopic examinations are particularly important in patients who have had progressive or constant hoarseness for more than 2 to 3 weeks, because this may indicate vocal fold lesion. Studies have linked the presence of LPR with upper aerodigestive tract cancers, especially in patients with additional risk factors, such as avid tobacco smoking and alcohol consumption.[19]

Voice disturbances

Many studies have investigated the most frequent symptoms and signs associated with LPR, one of the most consistent of which is voice disturbances. Specific examples of this include hoarseness, dysphonia, voice fatigue, and voice breaks. The symptoms have many physiologic bases, but usually these are associated with edema of the vocal cords, granulomas, or other vocal cord lesions. Furthermore, injuries related to trauma secondary to vocal abuse, endotracheal intubation, or upper respiratory infections may be slow to heal in patients with LPR secondary to repeated offenses by the refluxate.

Granulomas

When discovered, laryngeal granulomas should raise the clinical suspicion for LPR. However, numerous other potential causes of laryngeal granulomas exist, including smoking, chronic throat clearing and coughing, upper respiratory infection, vocal misuse, and trauma, such as intubation-related injuries. In a retrospective review of 55 patients with vocal cord granulomas, Havas and colleagues[20] found a 76% incidence of associated LPR or GERD based on laryngoscopic examinations or ambulatory 24-hour pH monitoring tests. The investigators also showed that the granulomas recurred in 50% of the patients who had surgical excision alone. Most patients who were treated medically showed resolution of granulomas. This finding is congruent with the current mainstay treatment plan of laryngeal granulomas, which is medical antireflux therapy along with correction of vocally abusive behaviors.

Laryngospasm

Laryngospasm is often paroxysmal, and is frequently associated with LPR. It most often occurs without warning, but some patients have described that the attacks occur in relation to certain activities, such as exercises and eating large meals. The direct stimulation of laryngeal sensory receptors by the refluxate or vagally mediated distal esophageal GER can cause partial or complete laryngospasm, which can be traumatic for patients. It can also be associated with bronchospasm, increased secretion, and tachycardia.

Laryngeal stenosis

Investigators have postulated and proven that LPR is a frequent cause of subglottic and posterior glottic stenosis.[3,21] LPR can cause significant and prolonged laryngeal inflammation. In animal models, intermittent acidic exposure to the subglottic region after mucosal injury has been shown to leads to nonhealing ulcerations and subglottic stenosis.[21] In humans, up to 92% of patients with subglottic stenosis were found to have LPR documented on pH studies.[3] In a more recent prospective case control study, Blumin and Johnston[22] showed that most patients (59%) with idiopathic subglottic stenosis had pepsin detected in the biopsies of their larynx and trachea. Combining aggressive antireflux therapy with precise surgery to relieve symptoms of laryngeal stenosis is a widely accepted and frequently successful treatment when LPR is suspected.

Laryngeal malignancies

The most critical risk factors for the development of laryngeal carcinoma are tobacco and alcohol use, which may have carcinogenic effect on the larynx. These factors also have the capacity to significantly influence patients' antireflux mechanism. They can decrease both LES and UES pressures, decrease mucosal resistance, increase gastric acid secretions, and even delay gastric emptying. In addition to tobacco and alcohol use, some studies have suggested that LPR plays a role in laryngeal malignancies. Kaufman[3] documented an 84% incidence of LPR in the 31 consecutive cases of laryngeal carcinoma, with only 58% being active smokers. Copper and colleagues[23] evaluated 24 patients with laryngeal and pharyngeal squamous cell carcinoma with a dual-probe pH study and determined that 11 had abnormal reflux confirmed on both probes and 4 had abnormal reflux on the proximal probe reading. More recently, Lewin and colleagues[24] conducted a study investigating the incidence of LPR in patients with early laryngeal carcinomas or premalignant lesions using objective data from a 24-hour pH monitoring and reflux area index. The study showed an 85% incidence of LPR in 40 patients with early cancer or premalignancy of the larynx. Although several studies have shown a reasonable link between LPR and laryngeal malignancies, investigators do not unanimously agree on this relationship. One of the latest studies investigating this relationship showed no direct association when more than

14,000 patients were retrospectively reviewed with adjusted tobacco and alcohol use.[25]

Diagnosis

Although the diagnosis of LPR has become more common in the past several years,[2] little progress has been made in the ability to confirm the association between the clinical manifestations and the underlying origin of reflux, making the institution of treatment problematic. Traditionally, otolaryngologists have considered resolution of symptoms with treatment of proton pump inhibitors (PPIs) to be diagnostic of LPR. Currently, the clinical diagnosis of LPR is established using several clinical tools along with a thorough review of patient histories.

Differential diagnosis

LPR is generally a chronic condition that results from repeated extraesophageal exposure to gastric refluxate. Other causes that lead to chronic laryngeal inflammation should be included in the differential diagnosis. If the patient presents with fever, fatigue, and an abrupt onset of symptoms, infectious origins need consideration. Infections can vary from bacterial infections, such as group A streptococcus and *Haemophilus influenza*, to viral infections, such as influenza, adenovirus, and rhinovirus. Acute laryngeal edema alone could be a result of an allergic or anaphylactic reaction. In more chronic forms of laryngitis, the differential should include autoimmune disease, granulomatous diseases, environmental injuries, and LPR. Autoimmune diseases that cause laryngitis generally have systemwide manifestation of symptoms. These conditions include rheumatoid arthritis, lupus erythematosus, and amyloidosis. Examples of granulomatous diseases include tuberculosis, scleroma, actinomycosis, leprosy, and syphilis. Fungal infections can manifest as granulomatous diseases in cases of candidiasis, blastomycosis, histoplasmosis, and aspergillosis.

Symptoms

Patients with LPR often lack classic symptoms of GERD, such as heartburn and regurgitation. Rather, patients display a constellation of extraesophageal symptoms, such as hoarseness, chronic cough, globus pharyngeus, dysphonia, sore throat, excessive throat clearing, and postnasal drip.

Belafsky and colleagues[26,27] developed the Reflux Symptom Index (RSI), which is designed to help diagnose patients with LPR. The RSI, presented in **Box 1**, is a scored self-administered survey that consists of nine questions. The investigators gathered normative data, which showed

---

Box 1
The Reflux Symptom Index

Within the past month, how did the following problems affect you? Rank them from 0 (no problem) to 5 (severe problem)

1. Hoarseness or a problem with your voice
2. Clearing your throat
3. Excess throat mucus or postnasal drip
4. Difficulty swallowing food, liquids, or pills
5. Coughing after you have eaten or after lying down
6. Breathing difficulties or choking episodes
7. Troublesome or annoying cough
8. Sensations of something sticking in your throat or a lump in your throat
9. Heartburn, chest pain, indigestion, or stomach acid coming up

From Belafsky PC, Postma GN, Koufman JA. Validity and reliability of the reflux symptom index (RSI). J Voice 2002;16(2):274–7; with permission.

---

that an RSI of more than 10 is associated with a high likelihood of LPR based on dual-probe pH study.[28] Furthermore, a prospective study of 40 patients with LPR who underwent 2 months of medical therapy showed significant improvement in the mean RSI from 19.3 to 13.9.[26]

Laryngoscopy

Laryngoscopy is a common screening tool for patients with symptoms such as hoarseness, cough, and laryngitis. Currently no single laryngoscopic finding is known to be pathognomonic to LPR. However, several laryngoscopic findings have been closely associated with LPR. One of these findings is pseudosulcus vocalis, which refers to infraglottic edema that passes posterior to the vocal process of the arytenoids cartilage. This pseudosulcus, as an independent laryngoscopic finding, has been strongly associated with LPR.[29,30] Another finding in LPR is ventricular obliteration, which refers to edema of the true and false vocal cords that appears to obscure visualization of the laryngeal ventricle. Interarytenoid mucosa and true vocal fold edema and erythema are perhaps the most specific findings of LPR.

Several studies have attempted to identify laryngoscopic features that correlate with treatment response. Park and colleagues[31] showed that significant improvement of posterior cricoids wall, arytenoid complex, and true vocal folds occurred after treatment with medical antireflux therapy. These investigators also found that symptomatic response was twice as likely if patients' laryngeal abnormalities involved the interarytenoid mucosa or vocal folds. A more specific analysis of the degree of laryngeal erythema using digitalization of video-documented laryngoscopy was performed to provide quantitative data on LPR-associated findings. This analysis showed that the color value for redness of the posterior laryngeal and vocal fold erythema in patients undergoing treatment for reflux laryngitis were significantly reduced over time and correlated with the clinical response to treatment.[32]

In a continued effort to devise a validated instrument to document the physical findings and severity of LPR, Belafsky and colleagues[29] also presented the Reflux Finding Score (RFS) in 2001. The RFS (**Box 2**) is a standardized scoring system that uses an eight-item clinical severity scores based on fiberoptic laryngoscopic examinations. It was designed to help clinicians better

diagnose LPR, evaluate clinical improvement, and assess therapeutic efficacy. The eight components of the scoring system include subglottic edema, ventricular obliteration, erythema, vocal fold edema, diffuse laryngeal edema, posterior commissure hypertrophy, granuloma, and excessive endolaryngeal mucus. RFS ranges from 0 (no abnormal findings) to a maximum of 26. The investigators noted that scores greater than 7 strongly correlated with LPR. Although RFS is starting to become a more widespread contributor in the diagnostic process for LPR, some concerns have been raised about its subjectivity and inter-rater variability.[33] In addition, some investigators contend that not all eight components should be equally weighed and associated with LPR, because some elements, such as true and false vocal fold edema, posterior cricoids erythema, and posterior commissure edema, may occur more frequently in patients with LPR. Nonetheless, in the investigator's validation study, the mean RFS for control subjects was 5.2, whereas the mean RFS for patients with LPR was 11.5. Findings showed that a patient with RFS of greater than 7 had LRP with a 95% certainty.[29]

Direct reflux monitoring

The gold standard for diagnosing and quantifying GERD is the 24-hour pH monitoring test. The study entails placing a thin catheter containing single or multiple electrodes in the esophagus. The most common technique involves distal probe placement at 5 cm above the LES. The probes are capable of sensing fluctuations in the pH between 2 and 7. For the duration of the test, the patient wears a data recorder that is connected to the probe. Patients keep a diary of events (eg, heartburn, cough, chest pain) and at the end of the study the pH tracing and the diary are compared to determine symptom correlation. Currently, the pH probe monitoring remains the most sensitive and specific diagnostic test available, and is the best way to confirm the presence of an abnormal amount of GER.

Although 24-hour pH monitoring can confirm GERD, it still does not link it with the presence of LPR. Some have used this technology to measure the proximal extent of reflux as a surrogate for detecting aspiration events. The first to study this was Patti and colleagues,[34,35] who performed dual-probe 24-hour pH monitoring studies on patients with chronic respiratory symptoms of unknown origin with the goal of identifying aspirating patients. In this study, aspiration was defined by respiratory symptoms that occurred within 3 minutes after a reflux episode detected by both proximal and distal pH probe. The idea

---

Box 2
The Reflux Finding Score

Pseudosulcus

0, absent; 2, present

Ventricular obliteration

0, none; 2, partial; 4, complete

Erythema/hyperemia

0, none; 2, arytenoids only; 4, diffuse

Vocal fold edema

0, none; 1, mild; 2, moderate; 3, severe; 4, polypoid

Diffuse laryngeal edema

0, none; 1, mild; 2, moderate; 3, severe; 4, obstructing

Posterior commissure hypertrophy

0, none; 1, mild; 2, moderate; 3, severe; 4, obstructing

Granuloma/granulation

0, absent; 2, present

Thick endolaryngeal mucus

0, absent; 2, present

RFS is a scoring system based on findings from laryngoscopic examination designed to help diagnose patients with LPR.

From Belafsky PC, Postma GN, Koufman JA. The validity and reliability of the reflux finding score (RFS). Laryngoscope 2001;111(8):1313–7; with permission.

is that if a lot of reflux reaches the proximal esophagus, some of it is more likely to cross the UES and become aspirated.

Building on this concept, others have measured pH in the pharynx as, theoretically, the closest approximation of aspiration. Oelschlager and colleagues[36] studied the value of using pharyngeal pH monitoring in combination with laryngoscopy to predict which patients had true LPR and would respond to GERD treatment. In the study, a four-sensor pH catheter was placed with the proximal sensor located 1.5 to 2 cm above the UES. To be considered an episode of pharyngeal reflux, the pH in the proximal sensor had to decrease to less than 4, drop more than one point from its previous baseline, and be accompanied by simultaneous drop in esophageal pH to less than 4 in all distal sensors. This study showed that when patients suspected of having LPR had laryngoscopic findings consistent with reflux and more than one episode of pharyngeal reflux, they were more likely to experience response to medical and surgical GERD treatment. Although correlating pharyngeal pH and aspiration makes a lot of sense, measuring pH in the pharynx has limitations. Reflux episodes may not be detected in the larger air-filled pharynx, and a reflux episode may be diluted and buffered, resulting in pH greater than 4. In addition, a high frequency of artifacts in the recordings occurs because of drying of the sensor and accumulation of mucus or foods on the sensor.

The Restech pH probe (respiratory Technology Corporation, San Diego, CA, USA) is a recent addition that attempts to overcome many of these difficulties associated with pharyngeal pH monitoring; it detects the presence of aerosolized acid and minute quantities of acid. The caliber of the probe is approximately 1 mm and its placement does not require endoscopy or manometry. The probe is placed intranasally, with the sensor in the pharynx and the guiding light-emitting diode light in the back of the throat. Its design and positioning allow the sensor to operate in the pharynx environment without drying out. Patients keep a diary of symptoms, which is later compared with the results from the data recorder. Azazi and colleagues[37] studied this new device in asymptomatic volunteers, and characterized normative and abnormal values. Validation studies of the thresholds and normal values from patients with LPR are underway to establish the efficacy of this device.

LPR symptoms may be elicited by a nonacidic component of the gastric refluxate. The gastric refluxate travelling retrograde usually gets more dilute and buffered by the time it reaches the larynx and the pharynx. It then stands to reason that aspiration events are frequently elicited by refluxate with pH higher than 4. For this reason, identification and quantification of nonacid refluxate is important in diagnosing LPR.

One of the latest additions to the diagnostic tools used for LPR is the combined multichannel intraluminal impedance and pH monitoring (MII-pH). This technique allows the detection of acid and nonacid reflux through its ability to identify the presence of GER independent of pH at different levels in the esophagus.[38]

With impedance testing, the changes in electrical conductance are detected using multiple impedance measuring sites along the esophageal lumen. When these conductance changes are tracked, the interpreter can determine the direction of fluid movement within the lumen of the esophagus. Addition of the pH monitoring to the impedance analysis can detect acid and nonacid reflux events. MII-pH has limitations, however. No established normative values exist for all parameters acquired during MII-pH. Profound differences exist in the general population with regard to nonacid reflux that depend on habits and lifestyles. For example, eating and drinking behavior and style will most certainly have influence on reflux and its contents. These widespread differences will be difficult to reconcile when establishing the normative values. Another limitation is the relative complexity in interpreting each study. The interanalyst variability has not yet been determined.

Treatment

When treating patients with LPR, providers should first identify and address which lifestyle changes must be made. These modifications can range from smoking cessation, to eating habit changes, to changes in voice use. When symptoms persist despite the lifestyle changes, patients should undergo medical treatment before considering surgical options.

Preventive/diet

Addressing the reversible daily lifestyle choices that patients make is critical to the management of LPR. Studies have shown that simple changes aimed at nocturnal reflux prevention alone can yield substantial improvements in patients with posterior laryngitis and chronic dysphonia.[39] The list of modifications is well established and includes raising the head of the bed and strict avoidance of eating within 3 hours of lying down. Other commonly recommended modifications include avoidance of tobacco products, alcohol, fried and fatty foods, caffeine, chocolate, and spicy foods. Researchers have reported data showing that the distal esophageal acid exposure is decreased when these modifications are made.[5] Therefore, these lifestyle modifications may make a difference for patients with LPR.

Medications

Historically, histamine type 2 receptor blockers (H2Bs) were first considered optimal medical therapy in treating GERD and LPR, because they reduce gastric acid secretion along with pepsin production. They now play more of an adjunctive role in the therapy for GERD and LPR. Hanson and colleagues[39] reported that 54% of symptomatic patients with chronic laryngitis suspected of having LPR showed relief after 6 weeks of behavioral modification and H2B therapy, with a 92% recurrence after cessation of therapy.

In the 1980s, PPIs were introduced in the United States as drugs that inhibit gastric acid secretion through targeting the hydrogen-potassium adenosine triphosphatase (ATPase) pump. These drugs were found to be more effective than H2Bs for the long-term reduction of gastric acid production and treatment of erosive reflux esophagitis.[40] A once-daily PPI regimen may prove to be adequate in controlling significant esophageal reflux, but in cases of LPR, the laryngeal mucosa often require 24-hour protection. Therefore, patients are started on a twice-daily maximal PPI dose to prevent further injury, allow mucosal healing, and permit maximal symptomatic relief.[31] Many patients experience symptomatic improvement after 2 months of therapy, and laryngeal examination will continue to improve up to 6 months after antireflux therapy. Belafsky and colleagues[26] reported that symptom improvement was noted with twice-daily PPI in approximately 50% of the patients with LPR at 2 months and up to 72% of the patients overall from 2 to 4 months after starting medication. In a recent double-blind, randomized, placebo-controlled study, Lam and colleagues[41] showed a significant improvement in RSI in the treatment group compared with the placebo group after 6 and 12 weeks of twice-daily PPI (rabeprazole) therapy.

The effectiveness of PPI therapy in patients with LPR is not without controversy. Several studies contend that the symptomatic improvement is largely from a placebo effect. A study in 30 patients with reflux laryngitis symptoms compared 40 mg of omeprazole therapy given twice daily with placebo over 2 months. The results showed that both groups experienced improvement with no significant difference in outcomes between the groups.[42] Another study in 35 patients compared 40 mg of pantoprazole given once daily for 12 weeks with placebo,[43] and yet another study in 21 patients compared 40 mg of the medication given twice daily for 12 weeks with placebo.[44] Both of these studies showed improvement in laryngitis symptom scores, but no significant differences between the treatment and placebo groups.

Clinical trials have failed to end the controversy, because the studies have had different inclusion criteria, did not stratify populations based on LPR severity, lacked adequate controls, and often used different dosages and durations of medical treatment. Despite this controversy, many patients who have objective data indicating LPR are treated with PPIs. This treatment should be highly individualized. Not every patient's refluxate are of equal constituents. Those who have primarily acid reflux to the laryngopharynx are likely to benefit more from PPI therapy than those whose reflux is mostly nonacid in nature. This observation again highlights the importance of diagnostics modalities that help correctly select patients who might experience a response to medical therapy, and those who should undergo other treatments, such as antireflux surgery.

Surgery

Historically, medical and surgical management has been more difficult for controlling extraesophageal symptoms than for typical reflux symptoms, such as heartburn and regurgitation. Antireflux surgery is usually a gastric fundoplication to create a new valve mechanism at the gastroesophageal junction to prevent gastroesophageal reflux. Many types of fundoplications exist but the most common is a Nissen fundoplication, which is usually performed laparoscopically. In this fundoplication, the fundus of the stomach is mobilized and the posterior aspect of the fundus is passed behind the esophagus. The wrap is created over a length of 2 to 3 cm. After approximation of the crura with permanent sutures, the wrap is anchored to the diaphragm. Several studies have investigated the efficacy of antireflux surgery in treating LPR symptoms. Allen and Anvari[45] described a 71% improvement at 5 years postoperatively in patients whose primary symptom was cough. Deveney and colleagues[46] found that 73% of patients with reflux-induced laryngeal inflammatory lesion and voice disorders had resolution of symptoms after Nissen fundoplication. Similarly, studies from the authors' institution found that laparoscopic antireflux surgery provided improved extraesophageal symptoms in approximately 70% of the patients, whereas typical GERD symptoms were relieved in 90% of patients.[47]

Future Directions

Pepsin

Pepsin may have an integral role in the pathophysiology of LPR. Analysis of pepsin in laryngeal samples is an intriguing possible addition to the diagnostic tools available for LPR, and its detection may be a direct and accurate tool in the workup of patients with LPR symptoms. Johnston and colleagues[48] showed that pepsin is absent in the laryngeal specimens of normal controls and often present in those of patients with clinically diagnosed LPR. The University of Washington recently completed a pilot study[49] in which preoperative and postoperative pepsin assays were conducted on nine consecutive patients with LPR who underwent laparoscopic antireflux surgery. These patients were referred by the University of Washington department of otolaryngology based on clinical symptoms and laryngoscopic examinations. Of the nine patients, pepsin was detected in eight preoperatively. In all eight of these patients, symptoms improved postoperatively based on a symptom questionnaire. In seven of these patients, pepsin could not be detected postoperatively and one had a significant decrease in the detected amount. The only patient who did not have pepsin detected in the biopsy preoperatively did not experience clinical improvement of LPR symptoms postoperatively, despite normalization of her pH study. This study showed that pepsin detection in laryngeal cells has the potential to be an accurate diagnostic marker and possibly a predictor of success in the treatment of patients with LPR.

Alginates

Liquid alginate has been used in the treatment of symptoms of reflux disease for many years. It has been used largely in combination with H2B or PPIs. Sodium alginate forms a mechanical antireflux barrier within the fundus of the stomach. A pilot study showed the effectiveness of Gaviscon (GlaxoSmithKline, Uxbridge, United Kingdom) in treating LPR. A randomized, controlled, single-center study involving 24 patients who received 10mL of liquid alginate four times daily showed significant improvements in RSI and RFS compared with the control group who did not receive any treatment.[50] This difference was noted at 2-month and 6-month assessments. However, the placebo effect of alginates is unknown because the trial was not controlled with placebo. Nonetheless, given this improvement, further evaluation of alginates in the management of LPR is warranted.

SUMMARY

Evaluating patients with extraesophageal symptoms of GERD and diagnosing LPR is a complex process. Understanding the pathophysiology for LPR is important in not only evaluating patients but also treating them. Unfortunately, a gold standard diagnostic test for this entity is still lacking. However, behind the multidisciplinary efforts, a considerable amount of advancements continue to be made in understanding the pathophysiology of the disease, discovering the wide spectrum of otolaryngologic disorders associated with LPR, and devising treatment plans appropriate for LPR.

REFERENCES

1. Sontag SJ. The medical management of reflux esophagitis. Role of antacids and acid inhibition. Gastroenterol Clin North Am 1990;19(3):683–712.
2. Altman KW, Prefuer N, Vaezi MF. A review of clinical practice guidelines for reflux disease: toward creating a clinical protocol for the otolaryngologist. Laryngoscope 2011;121(4):717–23.
3. Kaufman JA. The otolaryngologic manifestations of gastroesophageal reflux disease (GERD): a clinical investigation of 225 patients using ambulatory 24-hour pH monitoring and an experimental investigation of the role of acid and pepsin in the development of laryngeal injury. Laryngoscope 1991;101(4): 1–78.
4. Lang IM, Shaker R. Anatomy and physiology of the upper esophageal sphincter. Am J Med 1997; 103(5A):50S–5S.
5. Ulualp SO, Toohill RJ. Laryngopharyngeal reflux: state of the art diagnosis and treatment. Otolaryngol Clin North Am 2000;33(4):785–802.
6. Erickson E, Sivasankar M. Simulated reflux decreases vocal fold epithelial barrier resistance. Laryngoscope 2010;120(8):1569–75.
7. Hanson DG, Jiang JJ. Diagnosis and management of chronic laryngitis associated with reflux. Am J Med 2000;108(Suppl 4a):112S–9S.
8. Piper DW, Fenton BH. pH stability and activity curves of pepsin with special reference to their clinical importance. Gut 1965;6(5):506–8.
9. Johnston N, Dettmar PW, Lively MO, et al. Effect of pepsin on laryngeal stress protein (Sep70, Sep53, and Hsp70) response: role in laryngopharyngeal reflux disease. Ann Otol Rhinol Laryngol 2006; 115(1):47–58.
10. Johnston N, Wells CW, Blumin JH, et al. Receptor-mediated uptake of pepsin by laryngeal epithelial cells. Ann Otol Rhinol Laryngol 2007;116(12):934–8.
11. Samuels TL, Johnston N. Pepsin as a causal agent of inflammation during nonacidic reflux. Otolaryngol Head Neck Surg 2009;141(5):559–63.

12. Loughlin CJ, Koufman JA. Paroxysmal laryngo-spasm secondary to gastroesophageal reflux. Laryngoscope 1996;106(12):1502–5.

13. Bauman NM, Sandler AD, Schmidt C, et al. Reflex laryngospasm induced by stimulation of distal esophageal afferents. Laryngoscope 1994;104(2):209–14.

14. Sasaki CT, Suzuki M. Laryngeal spasm: a neurophysiologic redefinition. Ann Otol Rhinol Laryngol 1977;86(2):150–7.

15. Cherry J, Margulies SI. Contact ulcer of the larynx. Laryngoscope 1968;78(11):1937–40.

16. Book DT, Rhee JS, Toohill RJ, et al. Perspectives in laryngopharyngeal reflux: an international survey. Laryngoscope 2002;112(8):1399–406.

17. Ford CN. Evaluation and management of laryngopharyngeal reflux. JAMA 2005;294(12):1534–40.

18. Ylitalo R, Ramel S. Extraesophageal reflux in patients with contact granuloma: a prospective controlled study. Ann Otol Rhinol Laryngol 2002;111(5):441–6.

19. Morrison MD. Is chronic gastroesophageal reflux a causative factor in glottis carcinoma? Otolaryngol Head Neck Surg 1988;99(4):370–3.

20. Havas TE, Priestley J, Lowinger DS. A management strategy for vocal process granulomas. Laryngoscope 1999;109(2):301–6.

21. Little FB, Koufman JA, Kohut RI, et al. Effect of gastric acid on the pathogenesis of subglottic stenosis. Ann Otol Rhinol Laryngol 1985;94(5):516–9.

22. Blumin JH, Johnston N. Evidence of extraesophageal reflux in idiopathic subglottic stenosis. Laryngoscope 2011;121(6):1266–73.

23. Copper MP, Smit CF, Stanojcic LD, et al. High incidence of laryngopharyngeal reflux in patients with head and neck cancer. Laryngoscope 2000;110(6):1007–11.

24. Lewin JS, Gillenwater AM, Garrett JD, et al. Characterization of laryngopharyngeal reflux in patients with premalignant or early carcinomas of the larynx. Cancer 2003;97(4):1010–4.

25. Francis DO, Maynard C, Weymuller EA, et al. Reevaluation of gastroesophageal reflux disease as a risk factor for laryngeal cancer. Laryngoscope 2011;121(1):102–5.

26. Belafsky PC, Postma GN, Koufman JA. Laryngopharyngeal reflux symptoms improve before changes in physical findings. Laryngoscope 2001;111(6):979–81.

27. Belafsky PC, Postma GN, Amin MR, et al. Symptoms and findings of laryngopharyngeal reflux. Ear Nose Throat J 2002;81(9):10–3.

28. Belafsky PC, Postma GN, Koufman JA. The association between laryngeal pseudosulcus and laryngopharyngeal reflux. Otolaryngol Head Neck Surg 2002;126(6):649–52.

29. Belafsky PC, Postma GN, Koufman JA. The validity and reliability of the reflux finding score (RFS). Laryngoscope 2001;111(8):1313–7.

30. Hickson C, Simpson CB, Falcon R. Laryngeal pseudosulcus as a predictor of laryngopharyngeal reflux. Laryngoscope 2001;111(10):1742–5.

31. Park W, Kicks DM, Khandwala F, et al. Laryngopharyngeal reflux: prospective cohort study evaluating optimal dose of proton-pump inhibitor therapy and pretherapy predictors of response. Laryngoscope 2005;115(7):1230–8.

32. Hanson DG, Jiang J, Chi W. Quantitative color analysis of laryngeal erythema in chronic posterior laryngitis. J Voice 1998;12(1):78–83.

33. Kelchner LN, Horne J, Lee L, et al. Reliability of speech-language pathologist and otolaryngologist ratings of laryngeal signs of reflux in an asymptomatic population using the reflux finding score. J Voice 2007;21(1):92–100.

34. Patti MG, Debas HT, Pellegrini CA. Esophageal manometry and 24-hour pH monitoring in the diagnosis of pulmonary aspiration secondary to gastroesophageal reflux. Am J Surg 1992;163(4):401–6.

35. Patti MG, Debas HT, Pellegrini CA. Clinical and functional characterization of high gastroesophageal reflux. Am J Surg 1993;165(1):163–5.

36. Oelschlager BK, Eubanks TR, Maronian N, et al. Laryngoscopy and pharyngeal pH are complementary in the diagnosis of gastroesophageal-laryngeal reflux. J Gastrointest Surg 2002;6(2):189–94.

37. Ayazi S, Lipham JC, Hagen JA, et al. A new technique for measurement of pharyngeal pH: normal values and discriminating pH threshold. J Gastrointest Surg 2009;13(8):1422–9.

38. Agrawal A, Castell DO. Clinical importance of impedance measurements. J Clin Gastroenterol 2008;42(5):579–83.

39. Hanson DG, Conley D, Jiang J, et al. Role of esophageal pH recording in management of chronic laryngitis: an overview. Ann Otol Rhinol Laryngol Suppl 2000;184:4–9.

40. Harris RA, Kuppermann M, Richter JE. Proton pump inhibitors or histamine-2 receptor antagonists for the prevention of recurrences of erosive reflux esophagitis: a cost-effective analysis. Am J Gastroenterol 1997;92(12):2179–87.

41. Lam PK, Ng ML, Cheung TK, et al. Rabeprazole is effective in treating laryngopharyngeal reflux in a randomized placebo-controlled trial. Clin Gastroenterol Hepatol 2010;8(9):770–6.

42. Noordzij JP, Khidr A, Evans BA, et al. Evaluation of omeprazole in the treatment of reflux laryngitis: a prospective, placebo-controlled, randomized, double-blind study. Laryngoscope 2001;111(12):2147–51.

43. Wu JM, Koopman J, Harrell SP, et al. Double-blind, placebo-controlled trial with single-dose

pantoprazole for laryngopharyngeal reflux. Am J Gastroenterol 2006;101(9):1972–8.

44. Eherer AJ, Habermann W, Hammer HF, et al. Effect of pantoprazole on the course of reflux-associated laryngitis: a placebo-controlled double-blind cross-over study. Scand J Gastroenterol 2003;38(5):462–7.

45. Allen CJ, Anvari M. Does laparoscopic fundoplication provide long-term control of gastroesophageal reflux related cough? Surg Endosc 2004;18(4): 633–7.

46. Deveney CW, Benner K, Cohen J. Gastroesophageal reflux and laryngeal disease. Arch Surg 1993; 128(9):1021–5.

47. Oelschlager BK, Eubanks TR, Oleynikov D, et al. Symptomatic and physiologic outcomes after operative treatment for extraesophageal reflux. Surg Endosc 2002;16(7):1032–6.

48. Johnston N, Knight J, Dettmar PW, et al. Pepsin and carbonic anhydrase isoenzyme III as diagnostic markers for laryngopharyngeal reflux disease. Laryngoscope 2004;114(12):2129–34.

49. Wassenaar E, Johnston N, Merati A, et al. Pepsin detection in patients with laryngopharyngeal reflux before and after fundoplication. Surg Endosc, 2011. [Epub ahead of print].

50. McGlashan JA, Johnstone LM, Sykes J, et al. The value of a liquid alginate suspension (Gaviscon Advance) in the management of laryngopharyngeal reflux. Eur Arch Otorhinolaryngol 2009;266(2): 243–51.

Management of the Obese Patient with Gastroesophageal Reflux Disease

Kevin M. Reavis, MD[a,b,*]

KEYWORDS

- Morbid obesity • GERD • Reflux • Adjustable gastric band
- Sleeve gastrectomy • Roux-en-Y gastric bypass
- Biliopancreatic diversion

Obesity and gastroesophageal reflux disease (GERD) are 2 of the most common chronic diseases affecting our society. Although the cause and manifestations of each are different, they commonly coexist and, in many circumstances, are directly associated. With increasing body mass index (BMI; calculated in kg/m^2), there is a direct relationship with the prevalence of GERD. Intra-abdominal pressure in the obese patient correlates with the presence of a greater number of obesity-related comorbid conditions in general and obesity alone has been identified an independent risk factor for the development of GERD.[1,2] Increasing intra-abdominal pressure associated with increasing BMI induces dysfunction of the antireflux barrier created by the lower esophageal sphincter.[3,4] Crookes and colleagues analyzed 1659 patients and established a relationship between increasing BMI and the prevalence of GERD.[5] Increasing BMI was positively correlated with increasing esophageal acid exposure, and the prevalence of a defective lower esophageal sphincter was higher in patients with higher BMI. Compared with patients with normal weight, obese patients are more than twice as likely to have a mechanically defective lower esophageal sphincter.[5] The lack of this barrier allows for gastric contents to reflux into the esophagus causing the typical symptoms of heartburn,

dysphasia, and regurgitation.[6] The prevalence of GERD in Western nations ranges from 10% to 20% in the general population and the number of outpatient visits for GERD in the United States is increasing.[7] The prevalence of GERD is much higher in the obese patient population, with rates of GERD reported as high as 70% in those qualifying for bariatric surgery, making it one of the most common comorbid conditions in the obese patient.[3] Currently greater than 50% of the United States population is either overweight or obese, with more than 5% of the population qualifying for weight loss surgery, and the percentage increases each year. Along with GERD, these patients suffer comorbid conditions including diabetes, hypertension, osteoarthritis, dyslipidemia, and others affecting every major organ system in the body and ultimately resulting in shorter life expectancy than nonobese individuals.[8]

TREATMENT OF MILD TO MODERATE DISEASE

Obesity and GERD are treated according to severity. Lifestyle adjustments are used in mild cases, for example using a supervised diet and exercise regimen for obesity and avoiding certain foods as well as using favorable nighttime sleeping

Disclosure: The author has nothing to disclose.
[a] Division of Gastrointestinal Surgery, Department of Surgery, University of California, Irvine Medical Center, 333 City Boulevard West, Suite 850, Orange, CA 92868, USA
[b] Veterans Affairs Healthcare System Long Beach, Long Beach, CA, USA
* Division of Gastrointestinal Surgery, Department of Surgery, University of California, Irvine Medical Center, 333 City Boulevard West, Suite 850, Orange, CA 92868.
E-mail address: kreavis@uci.edu

Thorac Surg Clin 21 (2011) 489–498
doi:10.1016/j.thorsurg.2011.08.004
1547-4127/11/$ – see front matter © 2011 Published by Elsevier Inc.

positions to treat mild GERD. Medical intervention in the form of appetite suppression and metabolic enhancement for obesity and acid suppression and mucosal protection for GERD are used to treat moderate levels of each disease. Patients can lose 15% to 20% of excess body weight with carefully supervised diet and exercise, which is associated with lower rates of GERD; however, attempts at losing greater amounts of weight and effectively keeping it from returning during long-term follow-up has proved to be a difficult challenge. The medical treatment of moderate GERD in both normal BMI and obese patients is through antisecretory pharmaceuticals such as proton pump inhibitors, Histamine$_2$ blockers, and antacids. Proton pump inhibitors are considered to be the principle treatment of moderate GERD because of the prolonged symptom relief and increased rate of mucosal healing.[9,10] However, 30% to 40% of patients presenting with GERD are incompletely responsive to proton pump inhibitor therapy and 50% to 75% of patients have recurrence of symptoms if they cease the use of these medications.[11] This phenomenon is magnified in the obese population. Patients who receive little to no symptomatic relief or who do not wish to use long-term antisecretory medications can opt for a surgical intervention to potentially improve their quality of life.

PREOPERATIVE WORKUP

The preoperative workup of the obese patient with GERD involves coordinate evaluation of the patient's cause and potential treatment options for obesity in addition to the standard workup used for nonobese patients suffering with GERD. Regarding obesity, factors such as duration of obesity, former attempts at weight loss, and psychosocial factors (such as a fear of being thin or family dynamics resisting weight loss) must be determined and incorporated into the overall treatment plan. In addition, patients are considered candidates for bariatric surgery if they have a BMI equal to or greater than 35 kg/m^2 with at least 1 significant comorbid condition such as diabetes, hypertension, or dyslipidemia, or if they have a BMI equal to or greater than 40 kg/m^2 with or without comorbid conditions.[12] In confirming a diagnosis of GERD, the standard workup includes contrast esophagram, upper endoscopy, pH testing, and esophageal manometry, along with impedance testing to determine that the patient is a candidate for medical or surgical treatment of GERD and is not presenting with functional heartburn or other nonsurgical causes of GERD-like symptoms.

SURGICAL INTERVENTION

Surgical intervention in general is reserved for the most refractory cases of obesity and GERD. Restrictive, malabsorptive, or combination operations are used to treat severe obesity, and esophagogastric fundoplication or other forms of lower esophageal sphincter and valve reconstruction are used to treat severe GERD. Several of the bariatric operations used to treat severe obesity are also effective in concomitantly treating GERD (Table 1).[13] However, some may induce GERD. As the obesity epidemic continues to worsen in the Western world, surgeons who specialize in the surgical treatment of GERD will encounter an increasing number of patients who are also obese. The operative selection to effectively treat both conditions simultaneously is therefore of increasing importance.

ANTIREFLUX SURGERY

Currently, the laparoscopic Nissen fundoplication is considered to be the standard surgical treatment

Table 1
Antireflux and bariatric operations with comparative effects

Operation	Antireflux Barrier	Decreased Acid Secretion	Bile Diversion	Weight Loss
Fundoplication	Yes	No	No	No
Gastric banding	Yes	No	No	Yes
Sleeve gastrectomy	No	Yes	No	Yes
Roux-en-Y gastric bypass	No	Yes	Yes	Yes
Biliopancreatic diversion with duodenal switch	No	No	Yes	Yes

Data partially from Schauer P, Hamad G, Ikramuddin S. Surgical management of gastroesophageal reflux disease in obese patients. Semin Laparosc Surg 2001;8(4):256–64.

of medically refractory GERD, with 90% to 94% overall patient satisfaction and overall outcomes during long-term follow-up.[10,14–16] In patients with normal BMI, Nissen (360°) and Toupet (270°) fundoplications have proved to be successful in maintaining remission of GERD at 5 and 10 years after the index operation. The earliest reported 5-year and 10-year follow-up of laparoscopic Nissen and Toupet fundoplications revealed that 93% of the patients were free of significant reflux symptoms 5 years after surgery and, at 10 years after surgery, 89.5% of the patients were still free of significant reflux. The symptom-free status was higher following Nissen (93.3%) than Toupet (81.8%). However, both procedures resulted in respectable levels of GERD amelioration compared with similar patients being treated with medication (proton pump inhibitors) alone.[17] When these same procedures are performed in the morbidly obese patient for the control of GERD, the results are not as promising. The mechanism of action of a fundoplication involves creating a robust antireflux barrier; however, there is no reduction in acid secretion, bile diversion, or substantial weight loss (see **Table 1**). In a study following 224 patients for 3 years after a fundoplication, Perez and colleagues[18] noted a high recurrence rate after surgery in obese patients. The increasing recurrence rates correlated with an increasing BMI. Recurrent GERD was noted in 4.5% of patients with BMI less than 25, 8% recurrence for BMI 25 to 30, and 27% recurrence for BMI greater than 30. In contrast, another study following 194 patients for a mean of 3.2 years after Nissen fundoplication found that there was no correlation between increasing BMI and a poorer overall outcome regarding recurrence of GERD after dividing the patients into 3 groups: normal weight (BMI<25), overweight (BMI 25–29.9), and obese (BMI>30).[19]

In morbidly obese patients who undergo fundoplication for the treatment of medically refractory GERD, the long-term outcome is not clear. The index operation affects only the lower esophageal sphincter and esophagogastric junction without addressing comorbid conditions that serve as risk factors for the development of GERD, such as weight. The use of an operation that addresses GERD as well as weight-associated comorbid conditions in the obese patient may be required for long-term success.

BARIATRIC SURGERY

As opposed to reconstructing the esophagogastric valve for the treatment of GERD in morbidly obese patients, operations that affect reflux through other mechanisms have proved successful in this challenging patient population. Providing a mechanical barrier to reflux is important; however, operations that result in decreased gastric acid production, diversion of biliopancreatic juices, and those that induce weight loss all have potential roles in the treatment of GERD in this patient population (see **Table 1**).

Laparoscopic procedures such as adjustable gastric banding, sleeve gastrectomy, and Roux-en-Y gastric bypass have different antireflux mechanisms but also have proven efficacy in the treatment of GERD and result in significant reduction in weight and remission of comorbid conditions. Laparoscopic malabsorptive operations such as biliopancreatic diversion with duodenal switch have not been proved effective in the treatment of GERD.

ADJUSTABLE GASTRIC BANDING

The laparoscopic adjustable gastric band is technically the simplest of the bariatric procedures and is the second most commonly performed in the United States, behind the Roux-en-Y gastric bypass (**Fig. 1**). This procedure consists of the placement of an adjustable silicone gastric band immediately distal to the esophagogastric junction and imbricating the gastric fundus over the band

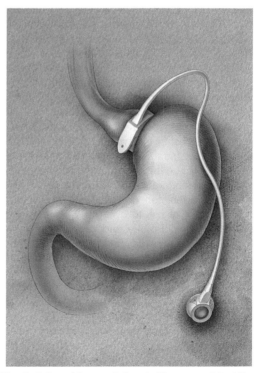

Fig. 1. Adjustable gastric band. (*Courtesy of* Covidien Surgical Services, New Haven, CT; with permission. Copyright © 2009 Covidien. All rights reserved.)

to secure it in place and create an approximately 15 cm^3 proximal gastric pouch. The band is then adjusted percutaneously via a subcutaneous port and intracorporeal tubing attached to the band. A Huber needle is used to access the port as needed and saline is injected (0–12 mL) to inflate the band and adjust gastric restriction. The adjustable gastric band is a purely restrictive operation. Because of its location on the proximal stomach, the band creates a theoretical barrier to reflux; however, it may induce reflux if it were to slip distally or if gastric pouch dilation occurs proximal to the band. It does not reduce gastric acid secretion or divert the flow of bile. It does induce significant weight loss (less than the sleeve gastrectomy and Roux-en-Y gastric bypass) and is associated with the resolution of GERD based on weight loss and its effect as an antireflux barrier (see **Table 1**).[13]

Many studies have found that adjustable gastric banding results in the amelioration of GERD. Dixon and O'Brien[20] reported 90% resolution or improvement in GERD in 48 patients who underwent laparoscopic gastric banding with a preoperative diagnosis of GERD. More recently, Brancatisano and colleagues[21] followed 838 patients (21% available for 3-year follow-up) after adjustable gastric banding and noted significant resolution in multiple obesity-related comorbidities. Excess body weight loss at 3 years was 54% (±23%; n = 175). In that study, there were 545 patients identified with comorbid illness at greater than 6-month follow-up. After a median follow-up of 13 months, resolution and/or improvement of type 2 diabetes mellitus was 79%; metabolic syndrome, 78%; hypertension, 67%; dyslipidemia, 66%; and gastroesophageal reflux, 66%. Quality of life was significantly improved as well. In contrast, Forsell and colleagues[22] followed 326 patients for a mean of 28 months (range 6–76 months) and noted GERD to be the most common complication not requiring reoperation (4.7%) after laparoscopic banding. The maintenance of normal esophageal motility is also at risk following the placement of gastric bands. O'Rourke and colleagues[23] conducted an animal study placing nonadjustable bands around the proximal stomach of opossums and followed them for 14 weeks. There was a 36% decrease in both baseline mean resting lower esophageal sphincter pressure and in the distal esophageal peristaltic pressure in banded animals. Motility disorders developed during the study in more than one-third of the banded animals. This phenomenon was observed in humans by Naef and colleagues[24] after 167 patients were followed for 73.8 (±6.8) months after undergoing adjustable gastric banding. Esophageal dysmotility

disorders were found in 108 patients (68.8% of patients followed) and esophageal dilatation occurred in 40 patients (25.5%). Although adjustable gastric banding has a potentially favorable track record regarding the resolution of GERD in humans, caution should be exercised regarding the overall effects of the induced gastric restriction on distal esophageal physiology.

SLEEVE GASTRECTOMY

The laparoscopic sleeve gastrectomy is more technically complex than the adjustable gastric band and is the newest of the bariatric procedures to gain acceptance by third party payers (**Fig. 2**). It consists of a stapled resection of the greater curve of the stomach initiated 2 to 6 cm proximal to the pylorus and proceeding cephalad to the angle of His. It is commonly performed over a 32 to 40 French bougie and serves as a restrictive operation with sleeve volumes approximating 50 to 80 cm^3. As an additional benefit of the resected greater curvature and gastric fundus, which serve as the source for the hunger-inducing hormone ghrelin, the sleeve gastrectomy also has a metabolic component and results in a sense of satiety after the operation. The esophagogastric junction

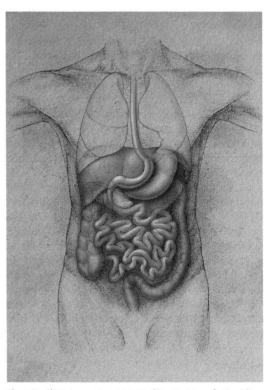

Fig. 2. Sleeve gastrectomy. (*Courtesy of* Covidien Surgical Services, New Haven, CT; with permission. Copyright © 2009 Covidien. All rights reserved.)

is left unaltered and thus no antireflux barrier is created. Because of the resected parietal cell–rich fundus and greater curvature, acid secretion within the tubularized stomach is decreased. Biliopancreatic juices are not diverted and significant weight loss is induced (less than the Roux-en-Y gastric bypass and more than the adjustable gastric band; see **Table 1**).

The mechanism of GERD resolution after sleeve gastrectomy is as much related to weight loss as it is to facets of the procedure itself. Typically, in morbidly obese patients who suffer from GERD with hiatal hernia, the concomitant correction of the hiatal hernia and sleeve gastrectomy reestablishes normal anatomic relationships and induces weight loss, which is associated with the resolution of GERD.[25] However, sleeve gastrectomy has also been implicated with both the treatment and development of GERD. Lazoura and colleagues[26] followed 85 patients for 1 year after sleeve gastrectomy. Radiographs were analyzed and 3 sleeve patterns were noticed, superior pouch (25.9%), tubular (65.9%), and inferior pouch (8.2%) patterns. Overall, patients showed a tendency toward relief of heartburn and increase of regurgitation and vomiting after surgery. However, only changes in regurgitation and vomiting were found to be associated with the tubular gastric pattern. Carter and colleagues[27] retrospectively analyzed 176 patients who had sleeve gastrectomy from January 2006 to August 2009. The average excess body weight loss at 6, 12, and 24 months was 54.2%, 60.7%, and 60.3%, respectively. Overall, 34.6% had preoperative GERD complaints. After surgery, 49% complained of immediate GERD symptoms, 47.2% had persistent GERD symptoms that lasted more than 1 month, and 33.8% of patients were taking medication specifically for GERD in the postoperative period. The most common symptoms were heartburn (46%), followed by heartburn combined with regurgitation (29.2%). Recently, Chiu and colleagues[28] conducted a systematic data search using Medline, EMBASE, the Cochrane Database, Scopus, and the gray literature for the keywords sleeve gastrectomy; gastroesophageal reflux; and equivalents. A total of 15 reports were retrieved. Two reports analyzed GERD as a primary outcome, and 13 included GERD as a secondary study outcome. Of the 15 studies, 4 showed an increase in GERD after sleeve gastrectomy, and 7 found reduced GERD prevalence after surgery. After completion of the systematic review, no consensus was reached regarding the effect of sleeve gastrectomy on the treatment or causation of GERD. Although sleeve gastrectomy successfully induces weight loss and many of these patients have some resolution of GERD, patients should be informed of the risks of GERD development, and this operation should be implemented with caution particularly in the morbidly obese patient with documented GERD in the preoperative setting.

ROUX-EN-Y GASTRIC BYPASS

The laparoscopic Roux-en-Y gastric bypass is more technically complex than the adjustable gastric band and sleeve gastrectomy, and is the most commonly performed bariatric procedure in the United States (**Fig. 3**). It consists of 3 components. By dividing the proximal stomach, a 30 cm^3 stomach pouch is created. A Roux limb is then created 40 cm (variable) beyond the ligament of Treitz and anastomosed to the gastric pouch. The proximal jejunal limb (biliopancreatic limb) is then anastomosed to the Roux limb 100 to 150 cm distal to the gastrojejunostomy. The small gastric pouch serves as the restrictive aspect of the operation and the bypass of the remnant stomach and proximal small bowel serves as

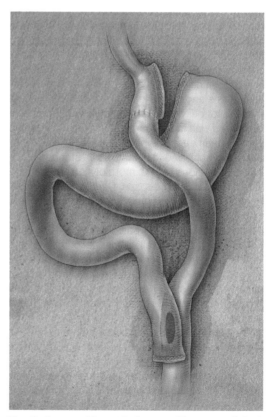

Fig. 3. Roux-en-Y gastric bypass. (*Courtesy of* Covidien Surgical Services, New Haven, CT; with permission. Copyright © 2009 Covidien. All rights reserved.)

the malabsorptive aspect of the operation. The esophagogastric junction is left unaltered and thus no antireflux barrier is created. Because of the proximal aspect of the gastric transection, acid exposure to the esophagus is nearly eliminated and acid secretion within the remnant is also decreased. The proximal stomach, where the pouch is created, has been shown to lack parietal cells and thus should produce minimal acid.[29] It has also been shown that basal and stimulated gastric acid secretion is virtually absent in the gastric pouch after gastric bypass.[30] Biliopancreatic juices are diverted and significant weight loss is induced (less than the biliopancreatic diversion and more than the adjustable gastric band and sleeve gastrectomy; see **Table 1**). Overall, the Roux-en-Y gastric bypass is considered to be the most reliable operation to treat severe GERD in the obese patient population.

Frezzi and colleagues[31] followed 152 morbidly obese patients with GERD for 12 months after Roux-en-Y gastric bypass. There was noted to be a significant decrease in heartburn (from 87% to 22%), water brash (from 18% to 7%), wheezing (from 40% to 5%), laryngitis (from 17% to 7%), and aspiration (from 19% to 2%). In these patients, the use of medication also decreased significantly regarding both proton pump inhibitor use (from 44% to 9%) and for histamine$_2$ blockade use (from 60% to 10%). SF-36 physical function scores and the mental component summary scores also revealed significant improvement after the operation. Jones and colleagues[32] also showed gastric bypass to be an effective antireflux procedure compared with fundoplication. Not only has gastric bypass been effective in treating GERD, but it has also been observed to be as safe as standard antireflux operations in the morbidly obese patient. Varela and colleagues[1] analyzed the University Health System Consortium database for patients who underwent laparoscopic fundoplication or laparoscopic gastric bypass from 2004 to 2007 (n = 27,264). The overall in-hospital complications were significantly lower in the laparoscopic gastric bypass group. Otherwise, the mean length of stay, observed mortality, risk-adjusted mortality, and hospital costs were comparable between the 2 treatment groups. In addition to safety observed with gastric bypass in the treatment of GERD, impressive prescription medication use and costs are reduced. Nguyen and colleagues[33] followed 77 morbidly obese patients for 1 year after gastric bypass. The mean excess body weight loss was 67% (±14%) 1 year after surgery. The mean number of prescription medications per patient was reduced from 2.4 before surgery to 0.2 1 year after surgery. The mean monthly medication

cost decreased from $196 before surgery to $54 1 month after surgery, representing a 72% cost saving. One month after surgery, the medication cost saving for GERD was 81%; for diabetes it was 69%; for dyslipidemia it was 53%; and for hypertension it was 43%. The mean monthly medication cost saving for the first year after surgery was $168 with a yearly savings of $2016 per patient. Improvement of GERD, diabetes, dyslipidemia, and hypertension was noted in this study to occur as early as 1 month after laparoscopic gastric bypass.

BILIOPANCREATIC DIVERSION WITH DUODENAL SWITCH

The laparoscopic biliopancreatic diversion with duodenal switch is the most technically complex of the bariatric procedures (**Fig. 4**). It is less often performed (<5% of bariatric operations in the United States) than the adjustable gastric band, sleeve gastrectomy and Roux-en-Y gastric bypass. It consists of 3 components. A conservative sleeve gastrectomy (larger than that of the

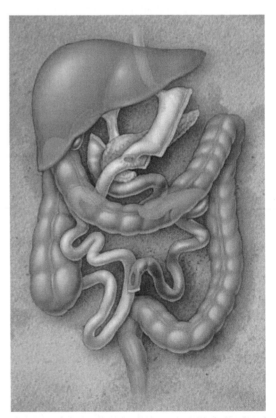

Fig. 4. Biliopancreatic diversion with duodenal switch. (*Courtesy of* Covidien Surgical Services, New Haven, CT; with permission. Copyright © 2009 Covidien. All rights reserved.)

stand-alone sleeve gastrectomy) from the angle of His to the gastric antrum is initially fashioned. The duodenum is then divided just beyond the first portion. A Roux limb is then created 40 cm (variable) beyond the ligament of Treitz and anastomosed to the proximal transected duodenum. The proximal jejunal limb (biliopancreatic limb) is then anastomosed to the Roux limb approximately 100 cm proximal to the terminal ileum. This configuration results in vagal and pyloric preservation, and eliminates duodenogastric reflux of biliopancreatic juices without vagotomy or gastric restriction. It is a predominately malabsorptive operation.

Despite being the most effective of the operations described for treating obesity, diabetes type 2, dyslipidemia, and hypertension, biliopancreatic diversion with duodenal switch has a less positive impact on the treatment of GERD in the obese compared with other operations. The esophagogastric antireflux barrier is unchanged after the operation and, because of the large amount of remaining functional stomach in these patients, gastric acid production is similar to that experienced in the preoperative state. Underlying this fact is the stomal ulcer rate of 8.3% to 12.5% observed in patients having biliopancreatic diversion with duodenal switch, which indirectly highlights the ineffectiveness of this operation in reducing acid secretion.[34] Biliopancreatic reflux is eliminated and, because patients with the biliopancreatic diversion with duodenal switch tend to lose the most weight of any of the bariatric operations, patients may have some improvement in GERD if the cause is primarily nonacid reflux and this is strongly influenced by the patients' obese body habitus (see **Table 1**). Overall, those patients with preoperative GERD have less resolution than those undergoing other bariatric operations such as adjustable gastric banding, sleeve gastrectomy, and Roux-en-Y gastric bypass. Prachand and colleagues[35] noted in their comparison of duodenal switch with Roux-en-Y gastric bypass that GERD resolution was greater in the gastric bypass group (76.9%) compared with the duodenal switch group (48.6%) 3 years after surgery.

TREATING REFRACTORY GERD AFTER BARIATRIC SURGERY

Although bariatric surgery is associated with amelioration or resolution of GERD in the obese patient, there are circumstances in which GERD persists. Therefore, alternative plans for these patients must be considered even before surgeons proceed with the initial operation. In mild cases, refractory GERD can be addressed in a similar fashion to when it presents initially, and can be treated with lifestyle adjustments and/or medication. In more severe cases, revisional surgery may be required.

Following adjustable gastric banding, well-known causes for the persistence or development of GERD include band slippage and proximal pouch dilation. For slippage, laparoscopically unbuckling the band and replacing it in the correct anatomic position (angled slightly up toward the left shoulder with a small gastric pouch on radiograph; **Fig. 5**) is often all that is needed to ameliorate the condition. When this is not adequate, removing the band along with conversion to Roux-en-Y gastric bypass is indicated to provide the patient with the best chance for definitive resolution of the GERD symptoms. More commonly than for refractory GERD, patients with adjustable gastric bands are converted to gastric bypass to address inadequate weight loss. Ardestani and colleagues[36] followed 19 patients requiring conversion of adjustable gastric band to gastric bypass because of inadequate weight loss or band erosion. Perioperative complications were acceptable, with 2 of 19 (10.5%) having surgical site infections without major intracorporeal complications.

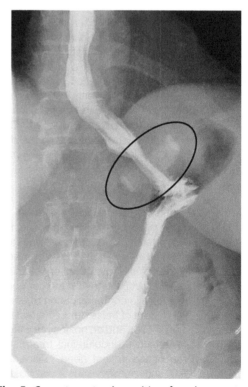

Fig. 5. Correct anatomic position for placement of adjustable gastric band.

As discussed earlier, sleeve gastrectomy has been credited for the resolution of GERD in some studies and implicated in the development of GERD in others. In patients who develop GERD secondary to distal stenosis near the incisura angularis, which can develop if the sleeve is made too narrow around this natural curve, opening the affected area via endoscopic dilation, distal gastroplasty (similar to a Heineke-Mikulicz pyloroplasty), or antrectomy with primary anastomosis can be performed.[24] Alternatively, the sleeve gastrectomy is designed to convert to Roux-en-Y gastric bypass, as an exit strategy for refractory GERD, by transecting the sleeve proximally and reconstructing with a Roux limb to provide the definitive treatment.[37]

Although Roux-en-Y gastric bypass is designed as a definitive antireflux operation in the morbidly obese patient, there are cases of refractory GERD. These cases can be caused by pouch dilation or a technical error resulting in a large pouch created at the time of the initial operation. If excessive acid exposure is present resulting in marginal ulceration of the proximal jejunum within the Roux limb, revision of the gastrojejunostomy (via resection and reanastomosis with a small gastric pouch) is warranted if medical management fails. If refractory GERD instead affects the distal esophagus and the pouch is of appropriate size, the situation is more challenging. A recent case series described using endoluminal radiofrequency energy to improve the robustness of the lower esophageal sphincter and antireflux mechanism. Mattar and colleagues[38] treated 7 patients a mean of 27 months after gastric bypass who had pH-confirmed GERD. Of the 7 patients, 5 patients had complete resolution of their symptoms, with normalization of pH studies. Follow-up was 20 (±2) months. One patient did not have adequate relief of symptoms after the treatment, and 1 patient was lost to follow-up.

EMERGING THERAPIES

The current standard for surgical treatment of GERD in the obese patient is the Roux-en-Y gastric bypass. Innovative technologies are pursuing new methods of treatment via an endoscopic approach. Currently, the 2 clinically available endoluminal treatments for GERD list BMI greater than or equal to 35 kg/m^2 as a relative contraindication to effective treatment.[39,40] Both of these devices affect the esophagogastric junction and do not induce weight loss. Therefore, effective endoluminal treatments of GERD in the obese patient need to address both the GERD and obesity issues, as do the more traditional surgical approaches. New endoluminal devices are being evaluated that act to restrict or divert food intake while excluding the stomach and duodenum, or that overlay the distal esophagus to effectively shield the various components of the foregut from one another.[41,42] No conclusive evidence exists that these devices are successful in long-term resolution of GERD or obesity; however it seems at this time that many investigative efforts are moving toward endoluminal treatments as an area of potential growth in this field.

SUMMARY

Obesity and GERD are 2 of the most common chronic diseases affecting our society. Although the cause and manifestations of each are different, they commonly coexist and require coordinate treatment. Only addressing GERD with an operation, while failing to address the other, often more serious co-morbid conditions associated with obesity, such as diabetes, hypertension, and dyslipidemia, is inadequate when treating the patient. Of the effective surgical treatments for GERD, fundoplication may be effective in the short-term control of GERD in the obese patient, but this procedure does not induce weight loss or treat comorbid conditions, and insufficient data exist to suggest long-term durability in this patient population. Of the bariatric procedures available, current evidence strongly supports Roux-en-Y gastric bypass as a highly effective treatment of GERD, obesity, and the associated comorbidities of obesity. Adjustable gastric banding and sleeve gastrectomy also treat GERD and induce weight loss, but both have been linked to the development of GERD as well, and potential conversion to gastric bypass must be considered at the time of operative decision making. The malabsorptive procedures have the least efficacy in treating GERD in the morbidly obese patient and should not be recommended for this purpose.

Patients with medically refractory GERD and a BMI greater than or equal to 35 kg/m^2 should consider Roux-en-Y gastric bypass if there are no other major contraindications to doing so. Adjustable gastric banding and sleeve gastrectomy should also be considered along with counseling of the patient regarding the potential need for conversion to gastric bypass. Surgeons who are not comfortable performing a bariatric surgical procedure should either complete appropriate advanced training in bariatric surgery or refer those patients to a qualified surgeon who can offer these options.

REFERENCES

1. Varela JE, Hinojosa MW, Nguyen NT. Laparoscopic fundoplication compared with laparoscopic gastric

bypass in morbidly obese patients with gastroesophageal reflux disease. Surg Obes Relat Dis 2009;5(2):139–43.

2. Ruhl CE, Everhart JE. Overweight, but not high dietary fat intake, increases risk of gastroesophageal reflux disease hospitalization: the NHANES I epidemiologic follow-up study. First National Health and Nutrition Examination Survey. Ann Epidemiol 1999;9:424–35.

3. Fisher BL, Pennathur A, Mutnick JL, et al. Obesity correlates with gastroesophageal reflux. Dig Dis Sci 1999;44:2290–4.

4. Mercer CD, Wren SF, DaCosta LR, et al. Lower esophageal sphincter pressure and gastroesophageal pressure gradients in excessively obese patients. J Med 1987;18:135–46.

5. Ayazi S, Hagen JA, Chan LS, et al. Obesity and gastroesophageal reflux: quantifying the association between body mass index, esophageal acid exposure, and lower esophageal sphincter status in a large series of patients with reflux symptoms. J Gastrointest Surg 2009;13(8):1440–7.

6. Locke GR III, Talley NJ, Fett SL, et al. Prevalence and clinical spectrum of gastroesophageal reflux: a population-based study in Olmsted County, Minnesota. Gastroenterology 1997;112:1448–56.

7. Friedenberg FK, Hanlon A, Vanar V, et al. Trends in gastroesophageal reflux disease as measured by the National Ambulatory Medical Care Survey. Dig Dis Sci 2010;55:1911–7.

8. Calle EE, Thun MJ, Petrelli JM, et al. Body-mass index and mortality in a prospective cohort of US adults. N Engl J Med 1999;341:1097–105.

9. Fock KM, Poh CH. Gastroesophageal reflux disease. J Gastroenterol 2010;45:808–15.

10. Dent J. Landmarks in the understanding and treatment of reflux disease. J Gastroenterol Hepatol 2009;24(Suppl 3):S5–14.

11. Cadière GB, Van Sante N, Graves JE, et al. Two-year results of a feasibility study on antireflux transoral incisionless fundoplication using EsophyX. Surg Endosc 2009;23:957–64.

12. Gastrointestinal surgery for severe obesity: National Institutes of Health Consensus Development Conference Statement. Am J Clin Nutr 1992;55(Suppl 2):615S–9S.

13. Schauer P, Hamad G, Ikramuddin S. Surgical management of gastroesophageal reflux disease in obese patients. Semin Laparosc Surg 2001;8(4):256–64.

14. Terry M, Smith CD, Branum GD, et al. Outcomes of laparoscopic fundoplication for gastroesophageal reflux disease and paraesophageal hernia. Surg Endosc 2001;15:691–9.

15. Lafullarde T, Watson DI, Jamieson GG, et al. Laparoscopic Nissen fundoplication: five-year results and beyond. Arch Surg 2001;136:180–4.

16. Hunter JG, Trus TL, Branum GD, et al. A physiologic approach to laparoscopic fundoplication for gastroesophageal reflux disease. Ann Surg 1996;223:673–87.

17. Dallemagne B, Weerts J, Markiewicz S, et al. Clinical results of laparoscopic fundoplication at ten years after surgery. Surg Endosc 2006;20:159–65.

18. Perez AR, Moncure AC, Rattner DW. Obesity is a major cause of failure for both transabdominal and transthoracic antireflux operations. Abstract 2109. Presented at the Society for Surgery of the Alimentary Tract, Digestive Disease Week. Orlando, FL, May 16–19, 1999.

19. Fraser J, Fraser J, Watson DI, et al. Obesity and its effect on outcome of laparoscopic Nissen fundoplication. Dis Esophagus 2001;14(1):50–3.

20. Dixon JB, O'Brien PE. Gastroesophageal reflux in obesity: the effect of lap-band placement. Obes Surg 1999;9:527–31.

21. Brancatisano A, Wahlroos S, Brancatisano R. Improvement in comorbid illness after placement of the Swedish Adjustable Gastric Band. Surg Obes Relat Dis 2008;4(3 Suppl):S39–46.

22. Forsell P, Hallerback B, Glise H, et al. Complications following Swedish adjustable gastric banding: a longterm follow-up. Obes Surg 1999;9:11–6.

23. O'Rourke RW, Seltman AK, Chang EY, et al. A model for gastric banding in the treatment of morbid obesity: the effect of chronic partial gastric outlet obstruction on esophageal physiology. Ann Surg 2006;244(5):723–33.

24. Naef M, Mouton WG, Naef U, et al. Esophageal dysmotility disorders after laparoscopic gastric banding–an underestimated complication. Ann Surg 2011;253(2):285–90.

25. Jossart G. Treatment of GERD after sleeve gastrectomy. (Oral presentation) American Society for Metabolic and Bariatric Surgery. Orlando, June 12–17, 2011.

26. Lazoura O, Zacharoulis D, Triantafyllidis G, et al. Symptoms of gastroesophageal reflux following laparoscopic sleeve gastrectomy are related to the final shape of the sleeve as depicted by radiology. Obes Surg 2011;21(3):295–9.

27. Carter PR, Leblanc KA, Hausmann MG, et al. Association between gastroesophageal reflux disease and laparoscopic sleeve gastrectomy. Surg Obes Relat Dis 2011. [Epub ahead of print].

28. Chiu S, Birch DW, Shi X, et al. Effect of sleeve gastrectomy on gastroesophageal reflux disease: a systematic review. Surg Obes Relat Dis 2011;7(4):510–5.

29. Berger EH. The distribution of parietal cells in the stomach: a histopographic study. Am J Anat 1934;54:87–114.

30. Smith CD, Herkes SB, Behrm KE, et al. Gastric acid secretion and vitamin B12 absorption after vertical

Roux en Y gastric by pass for morbid obesity. Ann Surg 1993;218:91–6.

31. Frezza EE, Ikramuddin S, Gourash W, et al. Symptomatic improvement in gastroesophageal reflux disease (GERD) following laparoscopic Roux-en-Y gastric bypass. Surg Endosc 2002;16(7):1027–31.

32. Jones KB, Allen TV, Manas KJ, et al. Roux-Y-gastric bypass: an effective antireflux procedure. Obes Surg 1991;1:295–8.

33. Nguyen NT, Varela JE, Sabio A, et al. Reduction in prescription medication costs after laparoscopic gastric bypass. Am Surg 2006;72(10):853–6.

34. Scopinaro N, Adami GF, Marinari GM, et al. Biliopancreatic diversion. World J Surg 1998;22:936–46.

35. Prachand VN, Ward M, Alverdy JC. Duodenal switch provides superior resolution of metabolic comorbidities independent of weight loss in the super-obese (BMI > or = 50 kg/m^2) compared with gastric bypass. J Gastrointest Surg 2010;14(2):211–20.

36. Ardestani A, Lautz DB, Tavakkolizadeh A. Band revision versus Roux-en-Y gastric bypass conversion as salvage operation after laparoscopic adjustable gastric banding. Surg Obes Relat Dis 2011;7(1):33–7.

37. Langer FB, Bohdjalian A, Shakeri-Leidenmühler S, et al. Conversion from sleeve gastrectomy to Roux-en-Y gastric bypass–indications and outcome. Obes Surg 2010;20(7):835–40.

38. Mattar SG, Qureshi F, Taylor D, et al. Treatment of refractory gastroesophageal reflux disease with radio-frequency energy (Stretta) in patients after Roux-en-Y gastric bypass. Surg Endosc 2006;20(6):850–4.

39. Available at: http://www.endogastricsolutions.com/esophyx_overview.htm. Accessed June 6, 2011.

40. Available at: http://www.mederitherapeutics.com/.

41. Available at: http://www.usgimedical.com/news/releases/20100915.htm. Accessed June 6, 2011.

42. Available at: http://clinicaltrials.gov/ct2/show/NCT01207804. Accessed June 6, 2011.

Diagnosis and Management of GERD Before and After Lung Transplantation

Toshitaka Hoppo, MD, PhD*, Blair A. Jobe, MD

KEYWORDS

- Gastroesophageal reflux disease • Lung transplant
- End-stage lung disease • Bronchiolitis obliterans syndrome

The strong association between gastroesophageal reflux disease (GERD) and the development and progression of pulmonary diseases has been suggested.[1–4] The progression of pulmonary diseases can lead to a need for lung transplant (LTx), which has been established as an accepted treatment strategy for selected patients with end-stage lung disease (ESLD). In the last decade, the short-term and long-term outcomes following LTx have been improving with the advance of surgical techniques and the refinement of immunosuppressive regimens and perioperative patient management.[5] However, the 5-year survival is approximately 50%, which has not changed in the past few years, mainly because of chronic allograft dysfunction caused by bronchiolitis obliterans syndrome (BOS). Because there has been no significant therapeutic impact on BOS in the last 20 years despite the use of novel immunosuppressive strategies,[6–8] the strong association between BOS and GERD has been suggested as a potential cause and thus a target for prevention and/or therapy.[8]

Accumulating evidence to support the association between GERD and ESLD would change the current algorithm for the management of patients with ESLD before and after LTx. Because GERD is curable, the proper management of underlying GERD would theoretically improve the outcomes. This article reviews the existing literature and the strategy to manage GERD in this population is discussed.

GERD AND ESLD

Since Belcher[9] initially summarized several case series, numerous reports have suggested the high prevalence of GERD in patients with diverse forms of lung diseases including idiopathic pulmonary fibrosis (IPF),[4,10–12] cystic fibrosis (CF),[1,13–15] chronic obstructive lung disease (COPD),[16,17] asthma,[18–21] and connective tissue diseases such as scleroderma.[22,23] The largest retrospective case-control study, involving more than 200,000 US veterans, showed that patients with erosive esophagitis as a sign of significant GERD had a 1.36 odds ratio (OR) of pulmonary fibrosis, a 1.28 OR of chronic bronchitis, and a 1.22 OR of COPD.[2] Although the pathophysiology of this association has not been well understood, it has been hypothesized that changes in diaphragmatic position (with compromise of the diaphragmatic pinch-cock action) and increase in positive intra-abdominal pressure and negative intrathoracic pressure (with a corresponding increase in the pressure gradient) may contribute to the development of GERD.[11]

Although the pathophysiology of IPF has been believed to involve aberrant fibroblast proliferation as a result of recurrent epithelial injury,[24] previous studies have shown that abnormal acid exposure in the distal esophagus was found in up to 88% of patients with IPF[4,11] and suggested that GERD may serve as a contributing factor to stimulate repetitive inflammatory reaction of airway and

Division of Thoracic and Foregut Surgery, Department of Cardiothoracic Surgery, University of Pittsburgh Medical Center, Suite 715, 5200 Centre Avenue, Pittsburgh, PA 15232, USA
* Corresponding author.
E-mail address: hoppot2@upmc.edu

Thorac Surg Clin 21 (2011) 499–510
doi:10.1016/j.thorsurg.2011.08.006
1547-4127/11/$ – see front matter © 2011 Elsevier Inc. All rights reserved.

pulmonary parenchyma for the pathogenesis and/or progression of IPF, especially for the acute exacerbation of IPF.[11] GERD is also common in patients with COPD, although less so than in patients with IPF. Previous studies have shown the association between the presence of GERD symptoms and increased frequency of COPD exacerbations[17] and indicated that decreases in esophageal pH were correlated with oxygen desaturation in nearly one-half of patients with GERD and COPD.[16] However, there are few reports regarding the prevalence of GERD in adult patients with CF. Small-cohort studies have shown the high prevalence of GERD in patients with CF (up to 91%),[1] and suggested that coexisting gastroparesis may be a significant contributing factor for GERD.[25] It is well known that scleroderma is associated with interstitial lung disease[23] and gastrointestinal tract dysfunction, especially esophageal motility disorder, which occurs in nearly all patients with scleroderma.[22] Common esophageal manifestations include severe esophageal motility disorder such as aperistaltic esophagus, esophagitis, and GERD, which has been considered a contributing factor in the pathogenesis of interstitial lung disease. In the recent prospective study involving 40 consecutive patients with scleroderma, Savarino and colleagues[23] showed that patients with pulmonary fibrosis (n = 18) had more frequent and higher reflux than those without pulmonary fibrosis (n = 22) and suggested that GERD could be responsible for the development of pulmonary fibrosis.

GERD AND LUNG TRANSPLANTATION

BOS is the leading cause of high mortality and morbidity after LTx and can occur at any time after LTx.[5] Obliterative bronchiolitis (OB) is distinguished pathologically by the compromise of small airways via lymphocytic infiltration and collagen deposition leading to luminal obliteration and progressive airway obstruction.[26] Because making the diagnosis of OB is challenging by means of transbronchial biopsy (sensitivity 28% and specificity 75%), BOS has been introduced as a clinical correlate for OB.[27] BOS characterizes the progressive decline in forced expiratory volume in 1 second (FEV_1) and the diagnosis of BOS is made based on a downward trend in pulmonary function criteria using FEV_1 and midexpiratory flow rate (FEF_{25-75}) as indirect measures.[27] Although the pathophysiology of BOS is not well understood, hypotheses of both alloantigen-dependent and alloantigen-independent mechanisms have been reported.[7,8,28–30] Because there has been no significant therapeutic impact on BOS in the last 20 years despite the use of novel immunosuppressive strategies,[8,31] GERD has been focused on as a potential alloantigen-independent cause and a target for prevention and/or therapy.[32]

Existing literature has shown that GERD after LTx is common, with up to 75% of patients having abnormal esophageal acid exposure and possible microaspiration as a cause of progressive lung damage,[33,34] repetitive acute rejection,[35,36] and BOS.[32,33] In patients who undergo LTx (post-LTx patients), the normal defense mechanisms against aspiration, such as cough reflexes and mucociliary clearance, of transplanted lungs are significantly impaired; for example, mucociliary clearance has been measured to be less than 15% of normal in transplanted lungs.[37] In addition, LTx seems to affect esophageal and gastric motility probably because of vagal nerve injury, ischemia, and local scarring related to surgery.[38] In the small prospective study involving 13 patients with lung malignancies undergoing major lung resection, Dougenis and colleagues[39] showed that pneumonectomy can cause esophageal and upper gastrointestinal dysmotility. D'Ovidio and colleagues[40] reported that delayed gastric emptying was found in 91% of post-LTx patients at 3 months and 81% at 12 months after LTx. The technical review by the American Gastroenterological Association stated that gastroparesis in lung transplant recipients predisposes to GERD with microaspiration.[41] Furthermore, the recent studies to evaluate an impact of bile acids on the transplanted lungs have shown an association between Pseudomonas colonization and the presence of bile acids in bronchoalveolar lavage, and suggested that epithelial defects by bile acids might predispose to colonization with Pseudomonas and airway neutrophilia, which potentially leads to BOS.[42,43] Despite these strong associations, the causal relationship between GERD and the development of BOS has yet to be definitively established.

EVALUATION OF GERD FOR PATIENTS WITH ESLD
Clinical Symptoms

Several studies have shown that typical GERD symptoms such as heartburn and regurgitation are not a reliable indicator of having pathologic GERD in patients with ESLD. In a cross-sectional study involving 512 patients with asthma or chronic bronchitis, Andersen and Jensen[44] showed that typical GERD symptoms had a diagnostic sensitivity of 89.5% and specificity of 47.1%. In another study involving 109 patients with ESLD awaiting LTx (pre-LTx patients), Sweet and colleagues[15] reported that symptoms were insensitive and nonspecific for diagnosing GERD (sensitivity 67%; specificity 26%) and that 33% of patients with distal reflux and 38% with proximal reflux were asymptomatic. Similarly, further studies for specific diseases such as COPD,[16] IPF,[4] and CF[1] supported the findings of low sensitivity and specificity of GERD symptoms.

However, atypical symptoms such as cough, hoarseness, dysphonia, globus sensation, and throat-clearing may be caused by direct gastric fluid exposure to the hypopharynx (direct mechanism) or vagal-mediated bronchoconstriction caused by gastric fluid exposure to the distal esophagus (indirect mechanism).[45] Laryngopharyngeal reflux (LPR) causes direct gastric fluid exposure to the hypopharynx.[46] In our series of 43 patients with ESLD,[47] 19 of 43 (44.2%) patients were minimally symptomatic or asymptomatic, whereas only 8 of 43 (18.6%) patients had purely typical GERD symptoms (heartburn and/or regurgitation). However, greater than 50% of patients had frequent LPR events, which were confirmed using multichannel intraluminal impedance pH with a specialized impedance catheter configured to directly measure LPR. Symptoms may be silent in patients with ESLD and objective esophageal testing is crucial for the proper management of GERD/LPR in this population.

Objective Esophageal Testing

The purpose of esophageal objective testing is to determine whether the patients' symptoms are caused by gastroesophageal reflux events, and to define the type of reflux and esophageal motility that will affect the selection of the surgical treatment options.

Barium esophagram

The purpose of barium esophagram is to evaluate the anatomy of the esophagus (ie, esophageal length) and to detect any organic abnormalities such as a hiatal hernia, mass lesion, and esophageal stricture. Although the presence of gastroesophageal reflux can be assessed during the study, the absence of radiographic evidence of reflux does not indicate the absence of GERD.

Upper endoscopy

Upper endoscopy is performed to examine the mucosa from the oropharynx to the second portion of the duodenum, and biopsies can be obtained if necessary. Mucosal disorders such as esophagitis, Barrett esophagus, and esophageal stricture are indicators for the presence of pathologic GERD. Nonerosive esophagitis is difficult to reliably recognize endoscopically and its presence may be confirmed based on the microscopic findings of mucosal infiltration with polymorphs, lymphocytes, eosinophils, and the recently described balloon cells.[46,48] Upper endoscopy may disclose unexpected findings such as malignancy, large hiatal hernia, and Zenker diverticulum. Abnormalities of the gastroesophageal flap valve can be assessed by retroflexion of the endoscope based on the Hill grading system.[49] The appearance of the valve correlates with the presence of increased esophageal acid exposure, occurring predominantly in patients with grade III and IV valves. Grade IV valve is compatible with a hiatal hernia.

Esophageal manometry

Manometry is an important component in the preoperative workup of patients who are candidates for antireflux surgery (ARS). The purpose of manometry is to exclude achalasia, which may be misdiagnosed as GERD, and to evaluate the degree of esophageal motility, based on which ARS may need to be tailored (Nissen or partial fundoplication). In addition, manometry allows the precise location of gastroesophageal junction (GEJ) to be measured for accurate pH probe placement. Although esophageal manometry used to be performed using water-perfused catheters with lateral side holes attached to transducers outside the body, high-resolution manometry (HRM) has been widely used with a solid-state manometric assembly with 36 circumferential sensors spaced at 1-cm intervals (outer diameter 4.2 mm) (Sierra Scientific Instruments Inc., Los Angeles, CA). HRM allows real-time monitoring of contractile activity for the entire esophageal length.

Biomarkers: pepsin and bile acids in bronchoalveolar lavage fluid

There has been accumulating evidence to support that biomarkers such as pepsin and bile acids in bronchoalveolar lavage fluid (BALF) could be useful to document the association between aspiration of gastric refluxate and lung injury and/or BOS. Ward and colleagues[50] showed that pepsin levels in BALF were measurable in post-LTx patients compared with no detectable pepsin in normal, nonsmoking controls, and proton pump inhibitor (PPI) therapy was not correlated with pepsin levels. This promising result led to a large prospective study involving 36 post-LTx patients, 4 normal volunteers, and 17 subjects with unexplained chronic cough to measure pepsin levels in BALF.[35] Pepsin levels in BALF were significantly higher in post-LTx patients and the highest levels were seen in post-LTx patients with acute rejection, a risk factor for progression to BOS.

On the other hand, post-LTx patients have an increased risk of duodenogastroesophageal reflux containing bile acids because of impaired foregut motility. D'Ovidio and colleagues[51] measured bile acid levels in BALF in 120 post-LTx patients with or without BOS to investigate its role in the development of BOS. Bile acid levels were increased in 20 of 120 (17%) patients, and bile acid levels in patients with BOS were significantly higher than in patients without BOS (1.6 mmol/L vs 0.3 mmol/L, respectively). In addition, bile acid levels correlated with BALF interleukin-8 and alveolar neutrophilia, both of which have been described as putative clinical markers of BOS development. Following this study, Blondeau and colleagues[52] further investigated the association between GERD and the degree of gastric aspiration in post-LTx patients with and without BOS using the combination of impedance testing and BALF testing for both pepsin and bile acids. Pepsin was detected in BALF of all post-LTx patients, whereas bile acids were detected in 50% of post-LTx patients. Post-LTx patients with BOS had neither increased GERD nor increased pepsin in BALF. However, 70% of patients with BOS had bile acids detected in BALF compared with 31% of stable patients. PPI did not reduce pepsin and bile acid levels in BALF. The investigators suggested that pepsin may be a more general marker of gastric aspiration, and that bile acids may be a more specific marker for BOS as an important pathophysiologic factor. In a further study, D'Ovidio and colleagues[40] investigated the impact of aspiration on pulmonary surfactant collectin proteins SP-A and SP-D and on surfactant phospholipids, all of which are important components of innate immunity in the lung, by performing dual-channel pH monitoring and BALF bile acid assay in 50 post-LTx patients 3 months after LTx. Abnormal pH findings were observed in 72% of patients who were positive for bile acids in BALF, and freedom from BOS was significantly reduced in patients with abnormal (proximal and/or distal) esophageal pH findings or BALF bile acids. In addition, pulmonary surfactant phospholipids and surfactant-associated proteins were significantly suppressed in patients with positive BALF bile acids and the investigators suggested that bile acids could promote BOS through direct epithelial injury or indirect dysregulation of lung surfactant proteins.

pH monitoring

Dual-channel pH monitoring with distal and proximal esophageal pH probes has been shown to be useful to evaluate patients with respiratory symptoms caused by proximal reflux events. Patti and colleagues[53] examined 70 consecutive patients with GERD symptoms using dual-channel pH monitoring (5 and 20 cm above the lower esophageal sphincter [LES]) and showed that patients with greater than 3% of acid exposure time in the proximal esophagus were more likely to have pulmonary aspiration. A further study from the same group showed that cough resolved in 19 of 23 (83%) patients after laparoscopic fundoplication when a correlation between cough and reflux was detected during pH monitoring, but in only 8 of 14 (57%) patients when no correlation was seen. In addition, cough resolved in 77% of patients who had a correlation between cough and acid exposure in the distal esophagus, whereas it resolved in 90% of patients who had a correlation between cough and acid exposure in both the distal and proximal esophagus.[54] This study indicated that acid exposure to the proximal esophagus is important for patients with respiratory symptoms and more sensitive evaluation in the proximal environment would lead to improved treatment outcomes.

Dual-channel 24-hour pH monitoring with esophageal and pharyngeal pH probes has been shown to be effective to evaluate patients with LPR.[55,56] In the study involving 518 patients with laryngeal or respiratory symptoms using combined esophageal and pharyngeal pH monitoring, Oelschlager and colleagues[57] showed that clinical history and individual symptoms cannot predict the presence of pharyngeal reflux, and that 43 of 181 (24%) patients with pharyngeal reflux had normal distal esophageal acid exposure, suggesting that conventional pH monitoring alone is not sufficient to detect patients with pharyngeal reflux. However, the pharyngeal pH probe is poorly sensitive secondary to pH probe drying and the relatively alkaline environment within the proximal aerodigestive tract. In addition, this testing is limited to measure acid LPR, not nonacid LPR, which also has caustic properties. A guideline of the American College of Gastroenterology stated that "available evidence does not support the routine use of proximal pH monitoring in clinical practice."[58]

Multichannel intraluminal impedance pH

Multichannel intraluminal impedance pH (MII-pH) is a new technology that enables the detection and measurement of intraesophageal bolus movement (regardless of pH) by detecting a change in resistance to current flow between 2 electrodes when a liquid and/or gas bolus bridges them.[59,60] When electrolyte-rich fluid is present between the 2 impedance electrodes, impedance decreases because of the flow of electrical current. In contrast, a gas event is poorly conductive and increases impedance. Based on these differences in impedance characteristics, liquid, gas, and mixed liquid-gas events can be differentiated. When multiple impedance electrode pairs are mounted on the same catheter, the direction and extent of bolus movement can be measured. An antegrade (proximal to distal) progression of impedance changes represents swallowing, whereas a retrograde (distal to proximal) progression represents a reflux event. Furthermore, the catheter configuration can be tailored by changing the location of impedance electrodes and pH probes based on the targeted reflux events.

Several studies have shown the potential benefit of MII-pH to evaluate patients with LPR[61-63] and that the proximal extent of reflux, rather than nonacid reflux, may play a more important role in the development of laryngeal symptoms.[61] However, the impedance catheters used in these studies were not optimized to directly measure LPR, because impedance electrode pairs and pH probes were mounted only in the esophagus (distal and proximal), not in the hypopharynx. Oelschlager and colleagues[64] used a specially designed bifurcated impedance catheter, in which one branch had 4 impedance electrode pairs in the esophagus with esophageal pH probe (5 cm proximal to the GEJ), and the other branch had a pharyngeal pH probe (2 cm proximal to the upper esophageal sphincter [UES]) with a pair of impedance electrodes distal and proximal to the UES. However, this catheter had only 1 pair of electrodes in the hypopharynx and it may have been difficult to differentiate pharyngeal reflux from the initiation of a swallow. Furthermore, a limitation to the implementation of hypopharyngeal impedance testing has been related to excessive noise secondary to air exposure and swallowing over the paired electrodes.

Recently, we developed a specialized, bifurcated impedance catheter configured to directly measure all forms of LPR (CZAI-B62C47E) (Sandhill Scientific, Inc., Highlands Ranch, CO, USA) (Fig. 1). The long-arm branch of the catheter had 2 electrode pairs in the distal esophagus with esophageal pH probe (5 cm proximal to the GEJ). The short-arm branch had 2 electrode pairs each in the proximal esophagus and the hypopharynx with the pharyngeal pH probe (0.5 cm proximal to the upper border of the cricopharyngeus muscle). In a prospective study involving 40 healthy volunteers to determine the normative data of LPR for 24-hour MII with this catheter, we showed that normal values of LPR were 0 off PPI and 1 on PPI.[65] Using MII with this impedance catheter to evaluate the pattern of reflux in 43 patients with ESLD (pre-LTx n = 19; post-LTx n = 24),[47] we showed that 56.3% of post-LTx

patients and 30.8% of pre-LTx patients had an abnormal number of LPR events (range, 1–8/d). However, a large number of patients had a normal number of total reflux events, which may have resulted in a negative DeMeester score. These data suggest that patients with ESLD have atypical patterns of reflux and conventional pH monitoring may not be sufficient to diagnose GERD in this population. Therefore, a direct measure of LPR is essential to guide treatment of patients with ESLD.

Gastric emptying study

LTx can cause gastroparesis, which predisposes to GERD with microaspiration. It is therefore important to evaluate the degree of gastroparesis in patients with ESLD. A gastric emptying study is performed with radionuclide-labeled meals (ie, eggs injected with technicium[99]) to assess emptying of solids and liquid. The gastric emptying half-time ($T_{1/2}$), defined as the time in minutes required for 50% of a radiolabeled meal to exit the stomach, is used to measure gastric motility. Patients with $T_{1/2}$ greater than 90 minutes are considered to have delayed gastric emptying. Previous studies suggested that patients with $T_{1/2}$ more than twice the upper limit of normal ($T_{1/2}$>180 minutes) should undergo pyloroplasty at the time of fundoplication.[66] However, the management of patients with $T_{1/2}$ between the upper limit of normal and twice the upper limit of normal (90–180 minutes) remains controversial.[67] Postoperative bloating can be treated by endoscopic dilation of the pylorus with botulinum toxin injection and a scheduled oral administration of simethicone. Recent case reports have suggested the potential benefit of gastric electrical stimulation for severe gastroparesis in this population.[68,69]

TREATMENT OF GERD FOR PATIENTS WITH ESLD
Medical Treatment: PPI, Macrolides

Acid suppression therapy using PPI and/or H_2 blockade has been widely used to treat GERD. Although acid suppression therapy is effective in controlling typical GERD symptoms, 35% to 40% of patients have recurrent GERD symptoms, probably caused by nonacid reflux.[70] Acid suppressive medications neutralize gastric acid but neither address the incompetence of LES nor stop reflux. This finding was confirmed by the study using MII-pH by Tamhankar and colleagues,[71] showing that PPI therapy does not affect the number of reflux episodes or their duration, and it converts acid reflux to nonacid reflux, thus leading to persistent symptoms and mucosal injury. In addition, previous studies using BALF biomarkers such as pepsin and bile acids have

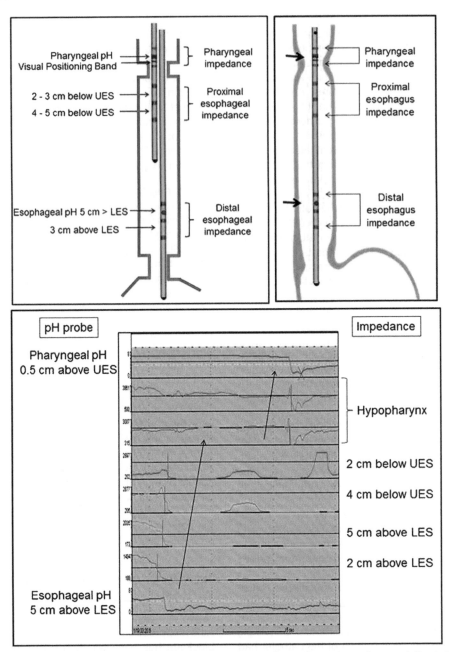

Fig. 1. Multichannel intraluminal impedance. (Upper left panel) Configuration of a specialized, bifurcated impedance catheter (CZAI-B62C47E). The long-arm branch of the catheter has 2 electrode pairs in the distal esophagus with the esophageal pH probe (5 cm proximal to the GEJ). The short-arm branch has 2 electrode pairs each in the proximal esophagus and the hypopharynx with the pharyngeal pH probe (0.5 cm proximal to the upper border of the cricopharyngeus muscle). (Upper right panel) Configuration of a single-arm branched impedance catheter (CZAI-BL-55). The catheter has the same configuration of bifurcated catheter. (Lower panel) Acid LPR confirmed using MII with this catheter. Esophageal pH drops to less than 4, followed by retrograde bolus movement that reaches the hypopharyngeal impedance, and then pharyngeal pH drops to less than 4. *From* Hoppo T. How much pharyngeal exposure is "normal?" Normative data for laryngopharyngeal reflux events using hypopharyngeal multichannel intraluminal impedance (HMII). J Gastroint Surg, in press; with permission.

shown that PPI therapy did not change pepsin and bile acid levels in BALF.[50,52] Although, PPI has been routinely used to treat GERD after LTx, there ~ has been no significant therapeutic impact

of PPI on the development of BOS in the past 20 years.

Given the increased prevalence of impaired gastrointestinal tract motility, medications that improve motility may have beneficial effect. Azithromycin (AZI) and erythromycin are macrolide antibiotics that have frequently been used in post-LTx patients in an attempt to prevent BOS. Macrolide antibiotics have been shown to increase the rate of total and proximal gastric emptying of both solids and liquids by producing a prokinetic effect on GI tract motility via activation of the motilin receptor.[72,73] Previous studies have suggested that AZI reduces gastric volume and modifies fundic acid distribution,[74] and also may reduce duodenopancreatic contest in the stomach by AZI-induced faster clearance of duodenogastroesophageal reflux from the stomach.[75] Several studies have suggested that AZI has a potential benefit for the prevention of BOS.[76–78] In the recent randomized controlled trial of AZI (n = 40) versus placebo (n = 43) in post-LTx patients,[79] Vos and colleagues showed that patients receiving AZI had less occurrence of BOS (12.5% vs 44.2%) and better BOS-free survival (hazard ratio 0.27) compared with patients on placebo during a follow-up of 2 years. However, overall survival, acute rejection, lymphocytic bronchiolitis, pneumonitis, pseudomonal airway colonization and GERD were comparable between groups. They concluded that AZI prophylaxis attenuates local and systemic inflammation, improves FEV_1, and reduces BOS 2 years after LTx.

Surgical Treatment

Since the first case report to show improvement in pulmonary function after fundoplication in a post-LTx patient was published in 2000,[6] several studies have shown that ARS potentially provides a survival benefit and delays the onset of BOS, particularly with early intervention (<90 days after LTx),[33,80] although the true benefit and optimal timing of ARS remain controversial. Davis and colleagues[33] reported that FEV_1 significantly improved by an average of 24% in 80% of post-LTx patients who underwent ARS (n = 43). The investigators suggested that it may be important to perform fundoplication before the late stages of BOS when irreversible fibrosis may be present, and hypothesized that early ARS may prevent BOS and improve survival. Based on this hypothesis, Cantu and colleagues[81] performed a retrospective review involving 76 post-LTx patients, in which survival was significantly better for patients who underwent early (<90 days) versus late fundoplication (100% vs 69%–86%; P = .03). Burton and colleagues[81] reported that fundoplication did not reverse any decline in lung function when performed at a mean time interval of 768 days (range 145–1524 days) after LTx in patients with

documented GERD. More recent data (abstract form) showed a 15.9% incidence of BOS in the early (<90 days) fundoplication group (n = 67) compared with 47.7% in the late group (n = 117) (P<.0001), although there was no significant difference in survival at 1 year follow-up between groups (97.0% vs 97.2%, P = .93).[82]

On the other hand, the use of ARS to preserve native lung function in patients with ESLD awaiting LTx (pre-LTx patients) should be considered because of the shortage of organs available for transplantation. However, the therapeutic benefit of ARS on ESLD progression has not been proved. Linden and colleagues[83] showed that 11 pre-LTx patients with IPF undergoing ARS had stabilization of oxygen requirement compared with other pre-LTx patients with IPF who did not undergo ARS at a median follow-up of 11 months. However, ARS did not significantly improve objective measurements of pulmonary function tests.

In a retrospective review of prospectively collected data involving 43 patients with ESLD (pre-LTx, n = 19; post-LTx, n = 24) at our institution,[47] we showed that FEV_1 improved in 91% of post-LTx and 85% of pre-LTx patients after ARS during a mean follow-up of 12 months. More importantly, of patients with declining FEV_1 before ARS, 92% of post-LTx and 88% of pre-LTx had a reversal of this trend after ARS. In addition, the pneumonia and acute rejection episodes were significantly reduced for post-LTx patients (both P = .03) and seemed to be stabilized for pre-LTx patients (P = .089). There was no correlation between the duration of time after LTx and responsiveness to ARS, even though all patients except 1 underwent ARS at greater than 90 days after LTx. Based on these data, ARS should be considered at any time point after LTx, and even more so if FEV_1 has declined. Because all patients were on antisecretory medication at the time of evaluation for GERD, these data support that a reconstruction of barrier function to reflux (ARS) is superior to acid suppression alone, and that the caustic effects of nonacid refluxate are likely related to lung injury via microaspiration.

TECHNIQUES OF ARS

A need for tailoring the type of ARS based on esophageal motility remains controversial. Recent randomized controlled trials have shown that the type of fundoplication needs not be altered in patients with ineffective esophageal motility who are not receiving transplants.[84–86] However, in our practice, laparoscopic Nissen fundoplication is the primary procedure for patients with normal esophageal motility, whereas laparoscopic Dor fundoplication is performed for patients with severe esophageal motility disorders defined by aperistaltic esophagus or greater than 50% failed swallows. Laparoscopic fundoplication is performed using a 5-port technique. The stomach is mobilized by dividing the short gastric vessels. A 3-cm length of tension-free intra-abdominal esophagus is obtained by extensive circumferential mediastinal dissection. The diaphragmatic crura are approximated with interrupted sutures and the fundoplication is created over a 60-Fr bougie. A 2.5-cm floppy Nissen fundoplication is performed with 3 stitches, incorporating the anterior esophageal wall. A satisfactory fundoplication is confirmed intraoperatively based on the endoscopic findings of a properly configured valve.[87] For patients with aperistaltic esophagus (scleroderma), we perform the modified Dor fundoplication, which includes reconstruction of the acute angle of His and anterior fundoplication with more than 15 fundus-to-crura sutures placed from the 4 to 9 o'clock positions over a 60-Fr bougie because of friable, edematous tissue.

PERIOPERATIVE CARE

Perioperative care is summarized in **Table 1**. Preoperative workup starts with the thorough review of medical records. Pre-LTx and post-LTx patients usually undergo the whole workup examinations including cardiac clearance (echocardiogram and cardioangiogram) and pulmonary

function tests. Because pulmonary hypertension is a contraindication of ARS before LTx in our practice, echocardiogram and cardioangiogram are essential to assess pulmonary arterial pressure in addition to the possible ischemia-related changes. Cardiopulmonary rehabilitation is critical to reduce the postoperative pulmonary complications and optimize the pulmonary function. The possibility of conversion to an open procedure should be discussed with the patients before ARS. Pre-LTx patients have little pulmonary reserve and should be counseled that an emergent LTx may be required should they develop perioperative pulmonary failure after ARS.

Patients are scheduled to stay in the intensive care unit overnight. Prophylactic anticoagulation in conjunction with sequential compression stockings is routinely performed to prevent deep vein thrombosis–related pulmonary embolism. Aggressive pulmonary toileting and early ambulation is routinely implemented to maximize the physical and pulmonary function. For post-LTx patients, a liquid form of immunosuppressive medication is started on the same day of surgery. Intravenous steroid is administered intraoperatively and postoperatively for patients with long-term steroid use. On postoperative day 1, a chest radiograph is obtained, a clear liquid diet is started, and patients are sent home from the intensive care unit if voiding, ambulatory, and without nausea. With any new increase in oxygen demand, patients should be kept in the hospital until this is treated

Table 1
Summary of perioperative care

Preoperative Care	Postoperative Care
Thorough review of medical records: assessment of functional status	DVT/PE prophylaxis, intravenous steroids for steroid cover, *Clostridium difficile* prophylaxis (probiotics), antiemesis
Esophageal objective testing	Intensive care as an immunocompromised host
Echocardiogram and/or cardioangiogram (r/o PH)	Aggressive pulmonary toileting and early ambulation
Pulmonary function tests	Immunosuppressive medications on day 0 CXR, clear liquid on day 1
Cardiopulmonary rehabilitation	Early discharge (on day 1 if voiding and ambulatory)
Discussion: conversion to open surgery, emergent LTx	Check tacrolimus level on day 2 if patients stay
Intraoperative Care	**Follow-up Instruction**
DVT/PE prophylaxis	Liquid diet for 1 wk, soft diet for 2 mo
Intravenous steroids for steroid cover	No heavy lifting >10 kg for 2 mo
Low procedure time	Follow-up at clinic at 2 and 6 wk

Abbreviations: CXR, chest radiograph; DVT, deep vein thrombosis; PE, pulmonary embolism; r/o PH, rule out pulmonary hypertension.

and resolved. Patients are instructed to follow a liquid diet for 1 week and a soft diet for 2 months, and to avoid heavy lifting (>10 kg) for 2 months. Patients are seen in the clinic at 2 and 6 weeks for follow-up. Postoperative diarrhea with or without *Clostridium difficile* is common, and can cause tacrolimus toxicity. Treatment with metronidazole should be started before the diagnosis is confirmed. In addition, all patients are placed on probiotics before surgery. All patients should be considered as an immunocompromised host, and strict hand washing and early discharge are emphasized to decrease exposure to pathogens. The tacrolimus level is highly variable and should be checked if patients cannot resume an appropriate oral intake the day following surgery. Patients with ESLD can have friable, edematous tissue because of long-term steroid use and immunosuppressive medications. It is important to consider that a prolonged tissue healing period is required, especially in patients requiring immunosuppression. The reduced gastric volume after fundoplication can lead to early satiety and may cause malnutrition in patients with CF who have pancreatic insufficiency and secondary malabsorption. A temporary feeding tube may need to be placed at the time of fundoplication in these patients. The benefit of surgical treatment of patients with scleroderma remains controversial.[22] In our experience, partial fundoplication (Dor) was successfully performed on 7 patients with scleroderma without any significant postoperative complications such as dysphagia. Most importantly, close communication with transplant pulmonologists and transplant surgeons is essential for the successful management of patients with ESLD.

PROPOSED STRATEGY

Based on existing data and our experience, we recommend that all patients with ESLD before and after LTx should undergo esophageal objective testing for the evaluation of GERD and LPR regardless of whether patients are symptomatic, because patients with ESLD have atypical patterns of reflux that may be entirely asymptomatic. Esophageal objective testing should include upper endoscopy, barium esophagram, HRM, MII-pH with a catheter configured to directly measure LPR, and gastric emptying study. Based on the normative data of LPR and full-column reflux (reflux to 2 cm below the UES) for MII-pH with a specialized impedance catheter configured to detect LPR, we constructed the proposed criteria of GERD and/or LPR in patients with ESLD (**Box 1**). GERD and/or LPR are considered present when LPR events (1 or more) were present on MII-

> **Box 1**
> **Proposed criteria of GERD and/or LPR in patients with ESLD using MII-pH**
>
> - LPR events ≥1/d on MII-pH
>
> or
>
> - Full-column reflux events ≥5/d on MII-pH
> - Plus any of the following signs:
>   - Esophagitis
>   - Barrett esophagus
>   - Hypotensive LES
>   - PPI dependence

pH or when full-column reflux events (5 or more) were present on MII-pH in addition to 1 of the following signs: (1) esophagitis (2) Barrett esophagus, (3) hypotensive LES, (4) PPI dependence.

All patients with ESLD who have documented GERD and/or LPR, especially with declining pulmonary function, should be considered ARS. For post-LTx patients, ARS should be considered at any time point when patients are stabilized and recovered from LTx. Our selection for pre-LTx ARS is individualized and is based on pulmonary function, functional status, and comorbid conditions. Patients with pulmonary hypertension are not candidates for ARS before LTx. It is critical to counsel that an emergent LTx may be required should they develop perioperative pulmonary failure after ARS because of limited pulmonary reserve.

SUMMARY

Although LTx is an accepted treatment strategy for patients with ESLD, the long-term survival remains limited mainly because of BOS. Accumulating evidence has shown a high prevalence of GERD in patients with ESLD and that GERD may play a role in the progression of ESLD and development of BOS as a causative or additive factor. Patients with ESLD have atypical patterns of reflux that may be entirely asymptomatic, and may have negative pH testing even if they have abnormal proximal reflux events such as LPR. There should be a low threshold for performing objective esophageal testing, including MII-pH (with a catheter configured to detect LPR) in patients with ESLD before and after LTx. To determine the true therapeutic benefit of ARS on patients with ESLD, a randomized controlled trial with long-term follow-up is required.

REFERENCES

1. Button BM, Roberts S, Kotsimbos TC, et al. Gastro-esophageal reflux (symptomatic and silent): a potentially significant problem in patients with cystic fibrosis before and after lung transplantation. J Heart Lung Transplant 2005;24(10):1522–9.

2. el-Serag HB, Sonnenberg A. Comorbid occurrence of laryngeal or pulmonary disease with esophagitis in United States military veterans. Gastroenterology 1997;113(3):755–60.

3. Napierkowski J, Wong RK. Extraesophageal manifestations of GERD. Am J Med Sci 2003;326(5):285–99.

4. Raghu G, Freudenberger TD, Yang S, et al. High prevalence of abnormal acid gastro-oesophageal reflux in idiopathic pulmonary fibrosis. Eur Respir J 2006;27(1):136–42.

5. Christie JD, Edwards LB, Kucheryavaya AY, et al. The Registry of the International Society for Heart and Lung Transplantation: twenty-seventh official adult lung and heart-lung transplant report–2010. J Heart Lung Transplant 2010;29(10):1104–18.

6. Palmer SM, Miralles AP, Howell DN, et al. Gastro-esophageal reflux as a reversible cause of allograft dysfunction after lung transplantation. Chest 2000;118(4):1214–7.

7. Riise GC, Williams A, Kjellstrom C, et al. Bronchiolitis obliterans syndrome in lung transplant recipients is associated with increased neutrophil activity and decreased antioxidant status in the lung. Eur Respir J 1998;12(1):82–8.

8. Shilling RA, Wilkes DS. Immunobiology of chronic lung allograft dysfunction: new insights from the bench and beyond. Am J Transplant 2009;9(8):1714–8.

9. Belcher JR. The pulmonary complications of dysphagia. Thorax 1949;4(1):44–56.

10. Salvioli B, Belmonte G, Stanghellini V, et al. Gastro-oesophageal reflux and interstitial lung disease. Dig Liver Dis 2006;38(12):879–84.

11. Tobin RW, Pope CE 2nd, Pellegrini CA, et al. Increased prevalence of gastroesophageal reflux in patients with idiopathic pulmonary fibrosis. Am J Respir Crit Care Med 1998;158(6):1804–8.

12. Sweet MP, Patti MG, Leard LE, et al. Gastroesophageal reflux in patients with idiopathic pulmonary fibrosis referred for lung transplantation. J Thorac Cardiovasc Surg 2007;133(4):1078–84.

13. D'Ovidio F, Singer LG, Hadjiliadis D, et al. Prevalence of gastroesophageal reflux in end-stage lung disease candidates for lung transplant. Ann Thorac Surg 2005;80(4):1254–60.

14. Ledson MJ, Tran J, Walshaw MJ. Prevalence and mechanisms of gastro-oesophageal reflux in adult cystic fibrosis patients. J R Soc Med 1998;91(1):7–9.

15. Sweet MP, Herbella FA, Leard L, et al. The prevalence of distal and proximal gastroesophageal reflux in patients awaiting lung transplantation. Ann Surg 2006;244(4):491–7.

16. Casanova C, Baudet JS, del Valle Velasco M, et al. Increased gastro-oesophageal reflux disease in patients with severe COPD. Eur Respir J 2004;23(6):841–5.

17. Rascon-Aguilar IE, Pamer M, Wludyka P, et al. Role of gastroesophageal reflux symptoms in exacerbations of COPD. Chest 2006;130(4):1096–101.

18. Harding SM, Guzzo MR, Richter JE. 24-h esophageal pH testing in asthmatics: respiratory symptom correlation with esophageal acid events. Chest 1999;115(3):654–9.

19. Harding SM, Guzzo MR, Richter JE. The prevalence of gastroesophageal reflux in asthma patients without reflux symptoms. Am J Respir Crit Care Med 2000;162(1):34–9.

20. Kiljander TO, Salomaa ER, Hietanen EK, et al. Gastroesophageal reflux in asthmatics: a double-blind, placebo-controlled crossover study with omeprazole. Chest 1999;116(5):1257–64.

21. Sontag SJ, O'Connell S, Khandelwal S, et al. Most asthmatics have gastroesophageal reflux with or without bronchodilator therapy. Gastroenterology 1990;99(3):613–20.

22. Ntoumazios SK, Voulgari PV, Potsis K, et al. Esophageal involvement in scleroderma: gastroesophageal reflux, the common problem. Semin Arthritis Rheum 2006;36(3):173–81.

23. Savarino E, Bazzica M, Zentilin P, et al. Gastroesophageal reflux and pulmonary fibrosis in scleroderma: a study using pH-impedance monitoring. Am J Respir Crit Care Med 2009;179(5):408–13.

24. Harari S, Caminati A. Idiopathic pulmonary fibrosis. Allergy 2005;60(4):421–35.

25. Bodet-Milin C, Querellou S, Oudoux A, et al. Delayed gastric emptying scintigraphy in cystic fibrosis patients before and after lung transplantation. J Heart Lung Transplant 2006;25(9):1077–83.

26. Stewart S. Pathology of lung transplantation. Semin Diagn Pathol 1992;9(3):210–9.

27. Estenne M, Maurer JR, Boehler A, et al. Bronchiolitis obliterans syndrome 2001: an update of the diagnostic criteria. J Heart Lung Transplant 2002;21(3):297–310.

28. DiGiovine B, Lynch JP 3rd, Martinez FJ, et al. Bronchoalveolar lavage neutrophilia is associated with obliterative bronchiolitis after lung transplantation: role of IL-8. J Immunol 1996;157(9):4194–202.

29. Verleden GM, Vos R, De Vleeschauwer SI, et al. Obliterative bronchiolitis following lung transplantation: from old to new concepts? Transpl Int 2009;22(8):771–9.

30. Snell GI, Westall GP. The contribution of airway ischemia and vascular remodelling to the

pathophysiology of bronchiolitis obliterans syndrome and chronic lung allograft dysfunction. Curr Opin Organ Transplant 2010;15(5):558–62.

31. Sato M, Keshavjee S. Bronchiolitis obliterans syndrome: alloimmune-dependent and -independent injury with aberrant tissue remodeling. Semin Thorac Cardiovasc Surg 2008;20(2):173–82.

32. D'Ovidio F, Keshavjee S. Gastroesophageal reflux and lung transplantation. Dis Esophagus 2006; 19(5):315–20.

33. Davis RD Jr, Lau CL, Eubanks S, et al. Improved lung allograft function after fundoplication in patients with gastroesophageal reflux disease undergoing lung transplantation. J Thorac Cardiovasc Surg 2003;125(3):533–42.

34. Hadjiliadis D, Duane Davis R, Steele MP, et al. Gastroesophageal reflux disease in lung transplant recipients. Clin Transplant 2003;17(4):363–8.

35. Stovold R, Forrest IA, Corris PA, et al. Pepsin, a biomarker of gastric aspiration in lung allografts: a putative association with rejection. Am J Respir Crit Care Med 2007;175(12):1298–303.

36. Shah N, Force SD, Mitchell PO, et al. Gastroesophageal reflux disease is associated with an increased rate of acute rejection in lung transplant allografts. Transplant Proc 2010;42(7):2702–6.

37. Herve P, Silbert D, Cerrina J, et al. Impairment of bronchial mucociliary clearance in long-term survivors of heart/lung and double-lung transplantation. The Paris-Sud Lung Transplant Group. Chest 1993; 103(1):59–63.

38. Suen HC, Hendrix H, Patterson GA. Special article: physiologic consequences of pneumonectomy. Consequences on the esophageal function. 1999. Chest Surg Clin N Am 2002;12(3):587–95.

39. Dougenis D, Morrit GN, Vagianos C, et al. Motility disorders of the esophagus before and after pneumonectomy for lung carcinoma. Eur Surg Res 1996;28(6):461–5.

40. D'Ovidio F, Mura M, Ridsdale R, et al. The effect of reflux and bile acid aspiration on the lung allograft and its surfactant and innate immunity molecules SP-A and SP-D. Am J Transplant 2006;6(8):1930–8.

41. Parkman HP, Hasler WL, Fisher RS. American Gastroenterological Association technical review on the diagnosis and treatment of gastroparesis. Gastroenterology 2004;127(5):1592–622.

42. Blondeau K, Mertens V, Vanaudenaerde BA, et al. Nocturnal weakly acidic reflux promotes aspiration of bile acids in lung transplant recipients. J Heart Lung Transplant 2009;28(2):141–8.

43. Vos R, Blondeau K, Vanaudenaerde BM, et al. Airway colonization and gastric aspiration after lung transplantation: do birds of a feather flock together? J Heart Lung Transplant 2008;27(8):843–9.

44. Andersen LI, Jensen G. Prevalence of benign oesophageal disease in the Danish population with special reference to pulmonary disease. J Intern Med 1989;225(6):393–402.

45. Lang IM, Haworth ST, Medda BK, et al. Airway responses to esophageal acidification. Am J Physiol Regul Integr Comp Physiol 2008;294(1):R211–9.

46. Barry DW, Vaezi MF. Laryngopharyngeal reflux: more questions than answers. Cleve Clin J Med 2010;77(5):327–34.

47. Hoppo T, Jarido V, Pennathur A, et al. Antireflux surgery preserves lung function in patients with GERD and end-stage lung disease before and after lung transplantation. Arch Surg, in press.

48. Narayani RI, Burton MP, Young GS. Utility of esophageal biopsy in the diagnosis of nonerosive reflux disease. Dis Esophagus 2003;16(3):187–92.

49. Hill LD, Kozarek RA, Kraemer SJ, et al. The gastroesophageal flap valve: in vitro and in vivo observations. Gastrointest Endosc 1996;44(5):541–7.

50. Ward C, Forrest IA, Brownlee IA, et al. Pepsin like activity in bronchoalveolar lavage fluid is suggestive of gastric aspiration in lung allografts. Thorax 2005;60(10):872–4.

51. D'Ovidio F, Mura M, Tsang M, et al. Bile acid aspiration and the development of bronchiolitis obliterans after lung transplantation. J Thorac Cardiovasc Surg 2005;129(5):1144–52.

52. Blondeau K, Mertens V, Vanaudenaerde BA, et al. Gastro-oesophageal reflux and gastric aspiration in lung transplant patients with or without chronic rejection. Eur Respir J 2008;31(4):707–13.

53. Patti MG, Debas HT, Pellegrini CA. Clinical and functional characterization of high gastroesophageal reflux. Am J Surg 1993;165(1):163–6 [discussion: 166–8].

54. Patti MG, Arcerito M, Tamburini A, et al. Effect of laparoscopic fundoplication on gastroesophageal reflux disease-induced respiratory symptoms. J Gastrointest Surg 2000;4(2):143–9.

55. Koufman JA, Aviv JE, Casiano RR, et al. Laryngopharyngeal reflux: position statement of the committee on speech, voice, and swallowing disorders of the American Academy of Otolaryngology-Head and Neck Surgery. Otolaryngol Head Neck Surg 2002;127(1):32–5.

56. Lee BE, Kim GH, Ryu DY, et al. Combined dual channel impedance/pH-metry in patients with suspected laryngopharyngeal reflux. J Neurogastroenterol Motil 2010;16(2):157–65.

57. Oelschlager BK, Chang L, Pope CE 2nd, et al. Typical GERD symptoms and esophageal pH monitoring are not enough to diagnose pharyngeal reflux. J Surg Res 2005;128(1):55–60.

58. Hirano I, Richter JE. ACG practice guidelines: esophageal reflux testing. Am J Gastroenterol 2007;102(3):668–85.

59. Fass J, Silny J, Braun J, et al. Measuring esophageal motility with a new intraluminal impedance device. First clinical results in reflux patients. Scand J Gastroenterol 1994;29(8):693–702.

60. Srinivasan R, Vela MF, Katz PO, et al. Esophageal function testing using multichannel intraluminal impedance. Am J Physiol Gastrointest Liver Physiol 2001;280(3):G457–62.

61. Anandasabapathy S, Jaffin BW. Multichannel intraluminal impedance in the evaluation of patients with persistent globus on proton pump inhibitor therapy. Ann Otol Rhinol Laryngol 2006;115(8):563–70.

62. Mainie I, Tutuian R, Agrawal A, et al. Combined multichannel intraluminal impedance-pH monitoring to select patients with persistent gastro-oesophageal reflux for laparoscopic Nissen fundoplication. Br J Surg 2006;93(12):1483–7.

63. Wu JC. Combined multichannel intraluminal impedance and pH monitoring for patients with suspected laryngopharyngeal reflux: is it ready to use? J Neurogastroenterol Motil 2010;16(2):108–9.

64. Oelschlager BK, Quiroga E, Isch JA, et al. Gastroesophageal and pharyngeal reflux detection using impedance and 24-hour pH monitoring in asymptomatic subjects: defining the normal environment. J Gastrointest Surg 2006;10(1):54–62.

65. Hoppo T, Sanz AF, Nason KS, et al. How much pharyngeal exposure is "normal?" Normative data for laryngopharyngeal reflux events using hypopharyngeal multichannel intraluminal impedance (HMII). J Gastrointest Surg 2011. [Epub ahead of print].

66. Farrell TM, Richardson WS, Halkar R, et al. Nissen fundoplication improves gastric motility in patients with delayed gastric emptying. Surg Endosc 2001; 15(3):271–4.

67. Van Sickle KR, McClusky DA, Swafford VA, et al. Delayed gastric emptying in patients undergoing antireflux surgery: analysis of a treatment algorithm. J Laparoendosc Adv Surg Tech A 2007;17(1):7–11.

68. Filichia LA, Cendan JC. Small case series of gastric stimulation for the management of transplant-induced gastroparesis. J Surg Res 2008;148(1):90–3.

69. Yiannopoulos A, Shafazand S, Ziedalski T, et al. Gastric pacing for severe gastroparesis in a heart-lung transplant recipient. J Heart Lung Transplant 2004;23(3):371–4.

70. Castell DO, Kahrilas PJ, Richter JE, et al. Esomeprazole (40 mg) compared with lansoprazole (30 mg) in the treatment of erosive esophagitis. Am J Gastroenterol 2002;97(3):575–83.

71. Tamhankar AP, Peters JH, Portale G, et al. Omeprazole does not reduce gastroesophageal reflux: new insights using multichannel intraluminal impedance technology. J Gastrointest Surg 2004;8(7):890–7 [discussion: 897–8].

72. Edelbroek MA, Horowitz M, Wishart JM, et al. Effects of erythromycin on gastric emptying, alcohol absorption and small intestinal transit in normal subjects. J Nucl Med 1993;34(4):582–8.

73. Peeters TL. Erythromycin and other macrolides as prokinetic agents. Gastroenterology 1993;105(6):1886–99.

74. Mertens V, Blondeau K, Pauwels A, et al. Azithromycin reduces gastroesophageal reflux and aspiration in lung transplant recipients. Dig Dis Sci 2009;54(5):972–9.

75. Koek GH, Vos R, Sifrim D, et al. Mechanisms underlying duodeno-gastric reflux in man. Neurogastroenterol Motil 2005;17(2):191–9.

76. Verleden GM, Dupont LJ. Azithromycin therapy for patients with bronchiolitis obliterans syndrome after lung transplantation. Transplantation 2004;77(9):1465–7.

77. Verleden GM, Vanaudenaerde BM, Dupont LJ, et al. Azithromycin reduces airway neutrophilia and interleukin-8 in patients with bronchiolitis obliterans syndrome. Am J Respir Crit Care Med 2006; 174(5):566–70.

78. Yates B, Murphy DM, Forrest IA, et al. Azithromycin reverses airflow obstruction in established bronchiolitis obliterans syndrome. Am J Respir Crit Care Med 2005;172(6):772–5.

79. Vos R, Vanaudenaerde BM, Verleden SE, et al. A randomised controlled trial of azithromycin to prevent chronic rejection after lung transplantation. Eur Respir J 2011;37(1):164–72.

80. Cantu E 3rd, Appel JZ 3rd, Hartwig MG, et al. J. Maxwell Chamberlain Memorial Paper. Early fundoplication prevents chronic allograft dysfunction in patients with gastroesophageal reflux disease. Ann Thorac Surg 2004;78(4):1142–51 [discussion: 1142–51].

81. Burton PR, Button B, Brown W, et al. Medium-term outcome of fundoplication after lung transplantation. Dis Esophagus 2009;22(8):642–8.

82. Balsara KP, Shah CR, Hussain M. Laparoscopic fundoplication for gastro-esophageal reflux disease: an 8 year experience. J Minim Access Surg 2008;4(4):99–103.

83. Linden PA, Gilbert RJ, Yeap BY, et al. Laparoscopic fundoplication in patients with end-stage lung disease awaiting transplantation. J Thorac Cardiovasc Surg 2006;131(2):438–46.

84. Booth MI, Stratford J, Jones L, et al. Randomized clinical trial of laparoscopic total (Nissen) versus posterior partial (Toupet) fundoplication for gastro-oesophageal reflux disease based on preoperative oesophageal manometry. Br J Surg 2008;95(1):57–63.

85. Robertson AG, Dunn LJ, Shenfine J, et al. Randomized clinical trial of laparoscopic total (Nissen) versus posterior partial (Toupet) fundoplication for gastro-oesophageal reflux disease based on preoperative oesophageal manometry (Br J Surg 2008; 95: 57–63). Br J Surg 2008;95(6):799 [author reply: 799–800].

86. Strate U, Emmermann A, Fibbe C, et al. Laparoscopic fundoplication: Nissen versus Toupet two-year outcome of a prospective randomized study of 200 patients regarding preoperative esophageal motility. Surg Endosc 2008;22(1):21–30.

87. Jobe BA, Kahrilas PJ, Vernon AH, et al. Endoscopic appraisal of the gastroesophageal valve after antireflux surgery. Am J Gastroenterol 2004; 99(2):233–43.

Management of Cricopharyngeal Dysphagia With and Without Zenker's Diverticulum

Brandon H. Tieu, MD[a],*, John G. Hunter, MD[b]

KEYWORDS

- Cricopharyngeus • Dysphagia • Zenker's diverticulum
- Diverticulum • Myotomy

Cricopharyngeal dysphagia is an abnormal sense of trouble swallowing solids or liquids through the upper esophageal sphincter (UES). Zenker's diverticulum (ZD) was described by Friedrich Albert Zenker, a German pathologist, in 1878.[1] A ZD represents an outpouching of hypopharyngeal mucosa through an area of muscular weakness between the transverse fibers of the cricopharyngeus (CP) muscle and oblique fibers of the lower inferior constrictors, known as Killian's triangle. ZD has a male predominance and occurs between the seventh and eighth decades of life. The prevalence within the general population is believed to be 0.01% to 0.11%[2]; however, the true prevalence may not be known because of a lack of reporting as regards asymptomatic ZD. The annual incidence of ZD has been estimated at 2 in 100,000 per year.[3] In this review, the authors cover the basic swallowing function, pathophysiology, and clinical presentation of cricopharyngeal dysphagia. In addition, the surgical and nonsurgical management of cricopharyngeal dysphagia with and without ZD is discussed.

ANATOMY, PHYSIOLOGY, AND PATHOLOGY

The UES is made up of the lower fibers of the inferior constrictor muscle, the CP muscle, and the upper part of the cervical esophagus (**Fig. 1**). The CP muscle is made up of horizontal and oblique fibers, and at rest is in a state of contraction. During normal swallowing, the CP muscle relaxes a fraction of a second before the arrival of an advancing bolus through the pharynx. In addition, the larynx elevates and moves anteriorly due to the contraction of the strap muscles, which then opens the CP muscle. After the bolus passes through the CP muscle and UES, the larynx descends and the CP closes and returns to a contracted state.[4] Inhibitory signals of a complex reflexogenic arc control the relaxation of the CP muscle, so disruption of this neurogenic process (eg, cerebrovascular accident, multiple sclerosis, amyotrophic lateral sclerosis) can result in failure of CP relaxation at the critical moment of bolus arrival.[5] Age-related changes have been noted in the swallowing mechanism, with delays in the initiation of the pharyngeal swallow, a decrease in the duration of the pharyngeal swallow, and a decrease in the opening duration of the CP. The anterior movement of the hyoid bone during swallowing is also delayed in elderly patients.[6]

There is no consensus regarding the pathogenesis of the ZD. It is theorized that the presence of an anatomic weakness of the posterior pharyngeal

The authors have nothing to disclose.
a Division of Cardiothoracic Surgery, Oregon Health & Sciences University, 3181 Southwest Sam Jackson Park Road, L223, Portland, OR 97239-3098, USA
b Department of Surgery, Oregon Health & Sciences University, 3181 Southwest Sam Jackson Park Road, L223, Portland, OR 97239-3098, USA
* Corresponding author.
E-mail address: tieub@ohsu.edu

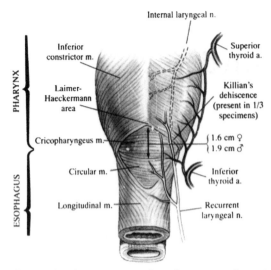

Fig. 1. Cricopharyngeus muscle and upper esophageal sphincter. a., artery; m., muscle; n., nerve. (*Reprinted from* Kelly JH. Management of upper esophageal sphincter disorders: indications and complications of myotomy. Am J Med 2000;108(Suppl 4a):43S–46S; with permission.)

musculature above the CP muscle and/or a muscular dysfunction of the UES predisposes to the formation of a ZD.[7] It has been proposed that excessive contraction of the CP or dyscoordination of contraction between the pharyngeal and CP muscles predisposes to herniation of pharyngeal mucosa, which has been termed the "neuromuscular dysfunction theory."[7] Another proposed theory is that gastroesophageal reflux can result in CP spasm and with an increased muscular tone may play a role in the development of ZD.[5] Manometric studies have had mixed results in their attempts to show increased contraction pressures or dyscoordination between the pharyngeal and UES muscles that would completely support these theories.[8] Using a combination of manometry and fluoroscopy (manufluorography) increased intrabolus pressures have been demonstrated, resulting from CP muscle spasm.[9] Histologic changes within the CP muscle can also affect UES pressures. It has been noted in CP specimens with ZD that there is increased fibrosis and collagen content, fatty replacement of muscle, and an increase in tonically active muscle fibers.[10–12] These changes can lead to increases in UES pressures either by CP muscle spasm or through fibrotic changes to the CP, further supporting its role in the development of ZD.

CLINICAL PRESENTATION AND DIAGNOSIS

Evaluation of patients with dysphagia starts out with a detailed history. The medical history may

help determine whether the symptoms are from metabolic, systemic, neurologic, or drug-related disorders.[13] Patients with CP spasm and ZD may present with a globus sensation, which is the sense of a foreign object in their throat, or the need to swallow multiple times for pharyngeal clearance. Others present following an aspiration event or with weight loss and nutritional deficiencies. Patients with ZD can present with symptoms of dysphagia, regurgitation of food, halitosis, episodes of aspiration, or chronic cough.

CP dysphagia and ZD can be diagnosed with modified barium swallow (MBS) or manufluorography. An MBS can identify structural causes of dysphagia such as webs, diverticula, strictures, or masses, and can evaluate for abnormal swallowing mechanics including aspiration. If a mass or suspected neoplasm is identified, endoscopic evaluation is warranted. With the MBS a cricopharyngeal bar can be observed on the lateral projection, suggestive of CP dysfunction (**Fig. 2**). This bar is a shelf of barium visible on the posterior column at the level of the cricoid cartilage that persists throughout swallowing. This finding can represent CP muscle spasm or impairment of muscle compliance.[14] Manufluorography allows for the correlation of anatomic structures during swallowing with the resulting intraluminal pressures. Furthermore, intrabolus pressures can be obtained, which act as an indirect measurement of UES compliance.[13] Electromyography (EMG) can also be used to evaluate the swallowing mechanism. EMG recordings can assess for synchronization of swallowing with contraction of inferior constrictor muscles and relaxation of the CP muscle, CP spasm, or a failure of the CP muscle to relax.[15] Overall, a combination of the patient's history (symptoms, medical conditions, or previous treatments) and the findings from diagnostic testing (cricopharyngeal bar, presence of a ZD, elevated intrabolus pressures, or a failure of CP relaxation) will guide treatment decisions.

NONSURGICAL MANAGEMENT
Balloon Dilatation and Botulinum Toxin Injection

There are few published reports on balloon catheter dilation for CP dysfunction or dysphagia.[16,17] In a small series, successful improvement of dysphagia was noted in 5 elderly patients with primary cricopharyngeal dysphagia, at a mean follow-up of 21 months.[16] This approach may be an attractive option for elderly patients with significant comorbidities, but there is insufficient evidence to suggest that this is a long-term treatment for the majority of patients with CP dysphagia.

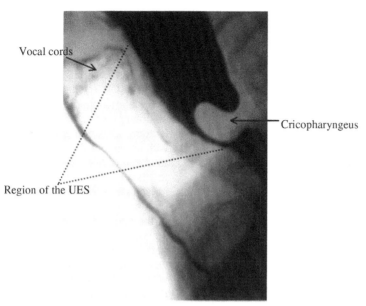

Vocal cords

Cricopharyngeus

Region of the UES

Fig. 2. Lateral image of a patient with a cricopharyngeal bar noted on barium swallow. UES, upper esophageal sphincter. (*Reprinted from* Sivarao DV, Goyal RK. Functional anatomy and physiology of the upper esophageal sphincter. Am J Med 2000;108(Suppl 4a):27S–37S; with permission.)

In 1994, the treatment of CP dysphagia with the injection of botulinum toxin (BT) A was reported in 7 patients.[18] Injection of BT can temporarily relieve dysphagia in patients who have isolated CP dysfunction or spasm by inhibiting its tonic and active contraction. The appeal of using BT is that it is minimally invasive with a low risk profile, and is less costly than surgery. Its main disadvantage is that if successful, it is only a temporary solution.[19] Others have suggested that a favorable response to BT may predict a successful outcome for surgical myotomy.[20,21] Its use in CP dysphagia has been reported in case series. Usually the procedure is done under general anesthesia under direct vision during transcervical surgery or endoscopic visualization. Injection of BT should be in the horizontal fibers of the CP muscle and not in the caudal fibers of the inferior pharyngeal constrictors. Complications include inadvertent pharyngeal or vocal cord injection with potential hoarseness or airway compromise.[22]

Transcutaneous injection of BT without sedation has also been described. Surface electrodes are placed on the chest and neck as a ground electrode and reference electrode, respectively, and connected to an EMG. After injecting local anesthetic, an injecting needle is used as the active monopolar electrode. Using EMG guidance, the needle is inserted near the inferior border of the cricoid cartilage, and is advanced posteromedially along the contour of the cricoid cartilage. Once insertion of the needle into the intrinsic laryngeal

musculature, the sternocleidomastoid or strap muscles has been ruled out, BT is injected into the inferior constrictor, CP, and upper esophageal musculature. In 13 patients with dysphagia treated with this technique for UES dysfunction and aspiration risk, 12 of 13 showed improvement in their ability to safely take an oral diet. Nine resumed a normal oral diet without the need for supplementation with a percutaneous gastrostomy tube.[23]

A systematic review of 12 reported case series in 2006 revealed 100 patients with oropharyngeal dysphagia who were treated with BT A. The etiology of dysphagia included central and peripheral neurologic causes, postsurgical swallowing derangements, and other diverse causes. Reported success rates varied from 20% to 100% with only 7 reported complications from the injection of BT. Six of the 12 studies reported a 100% success rate.[22] Proposed predictors of successful BT injection are those patients with less damaged swallowing function on videofluoroscopy and CP spasm based on EMG.[19] Potential reasons for BT A to fail to relieve dysphagia are a lack of standard method and dose for injection into the CP muscle, individual resistance to BT A, or structural changes to the CP muscle that render the BT less effective because of increased connective tissue and lower muscle fiber content.[19]

There is currently a lack of evidence to support the routine use of balloon dilatation or BT for the treatment CP dysphagia. These treatment options may be considered in a small subset of elderly patients with primary CP dysphagia who cannot undergo surgery, or as a predictor of success for surgical myotomy.

SURGICAL MANAGEMENT
Cricopharyngeal Myotomy

The first CP myotomy was described in 1951.[24] Endoscopic CP myotomy was first performed in 1994 using a potassium-titanyl-phosphate (KTP) laser.[25] Factors that favor a successful outcome for surgery include intact swallowing initiation, adequate laryngeal/hyoid elevation and pharyngeal propulsion with swallowing, and radiographic or manometric evidence of failed relaxation of the CP muscle.[13]

The open technique for CP myotomy is usually performed through a left cervical incision, but can be approached from either side of the neck. The sternocleidomastoid muscle is retracted laterally and the omohyoid muscle can be either retracted or divided. While retracting the carotid sheath posterolaterally, the larynx is rotated anteromedially to expose the pharynx and upper esophagus. The CP muscle is then divided down to the mucosa and carried cephalad for several centimeters above the esophagus. Complications from this approach include hemorrhage, recurrent laryngeal nerve injury, and fistulization of the pharynx or esophagus.

With the traditional endoscopic approach, the patient is under general anesthesia with the head placed in slight hyperextension. The specially designed endoscope or diverticuloscope is introduced into the proximal esophagus. The larynx is then lifted to expose the CP muscle posteriorly. The CP is then divided in the midline down to the prevertebral fatty tissue. This procedure can be done using electrocautery,[26,27] carbon dioxide (CO_2) laser,[28] or KTP laser.[29] In the absence of a ZD, the use of an endoscopic stapling device is not possible because the CP cannot be gripped posteriorly by the stapler. In a small series of patients, the CO_2 laser technique (14 patients) was compared with open CP myotomy (8 patients). Patients with ZD were excluded. The endoscopically treated patients had shorter operative times and hospital stays while achieving a similar success rate in functional swallowing to the open group. Overall complication rates were similar, but 2 patients in the open group had major complications. One had prolonged intubation and needed a tracheostomy because of medical comorbidities, and the other developed a pharyngocutaneous fistula.[30]

Management of Zenker's Diverticulum

Surgery remains the definitive treatment for ZD. Although the exact pathogenesis of ZD is still debated, most surgeons now believe that effective management of ZD involves the division of the CP muscle to break the muscle spasm thought to be primarily responsible for dysphagia. It was recognized in 1966 that CP myotomy was needed to address CP dysfunction associated with ZD.[31] Surgical management of ZD was initially done as an open procedure and involved either a diverticulectomy, diverticulopexy, or diverticular inversion with or without CP myotomy. For diverticulopexy, the base of the diverticular sac is fixed superiorly to the prevertebral fascia or the pharyngeal musculature. Inversion of the sac is performed by placing a purse-string suture around the neck of the sac and inverting the sac through it as the suture is tightly secured. These maneuvers eliminate the accumulation of debris within the sac. Open diverticulectomy was originally performed with hand-sewn repairs after resection of the diverticulum. This repair can be difficult deep down in the neck. Pharyngeal leaks and the development of mediastinitis was a concern with this technique. With the introduction of stapling devices, surgeons are able to perform sac excision and pharyngeal closure in a single step.[32,33] Bonavina and colleagues[34] reported 2 leaks in 116 patients (1.7%) treated with stapled diverticulectomy and CP myotomy. Both leaks were treated conservatively and healed within 2 weeks. Ninety-four percent of patients reported being symptom-free or significantly improved after a median follow-up of 48 months.

In 1917, endoscopic diverticulostomy was first performed by sharply dividing the common wall between the diverticulum and the esophagus.[35] This technique was popularized in 1960 in a report of 100 patients who were treated using diathermic coagulation, without any deaths or major complications.[36] Various sutureless techniques have been described, including the use of CO_2 lasers,[28] KTP/532 laser,[29] and electrocautery[26,27] using both rigid and flexible endoscopy. These techniques rely only on coagulation to seal the edges of the mucosa to prevent leakage and mediastinitis. The endoscopic technique has been extended with the use of ultrasonographic energy to coagulate and seal the tissue before it is divided. In a small study of 25 patients using this technique, the complication rate was 20% but no cases of hemorrhage, perforation, mediastinitis, or death were reported. Only 1 of 25 patients developed a recurrent diverticulum.[37] A modified technique of CP myotomy and resection of diverticula in patients with small (<3 cm) ZD has been supported by suture repair of the mucosa.[38] After sharply dividing the mucosa, the underlying CP muscle is divided using an insulated cannula coagulation device. Once the CP muscle has been divided, the mucosa is repaired with interrupted fine absorbable sutures. If a short ZD is present, the sac is everted into the laryngoscope with a cup grasper, and the mucosa is resected to remove part of the sac and expose the CP muscle. Once again the muscle is divided and the mucosa repaired. Using this technique, a small cases series of 14 patients was reported. In 12 of 14 dysphagia was completely resolved, but 2 patients persisted with mild dysphagia. If the patients tolerated their secretions on the day of surgery, they were started on a puréed diet the following day and discharged to home. This series did not report the length of follow-up, so it is unclear whether this procedure will provide durable, long-term relief of dysphagia.[38] Similar success was reported in 7 patients using a CO_2 laser with primary mucosal repair, without evidence of pneumomediastinum or mediastinitis. Two of these patients had a small cricopharyngeal bar (<1.5 cm ZD) while the rest had a prominent cricopharyngeal bar on MBS.[39]

In 1993, two surgical groups working independently were the first to describe using an endoscopic stapler to perform an esophagodiverticulostomy (ESD).[40,41] Due to the length of the stapling device and concern for incomplete division of the CP muscle, treatment of ZD smaller than 3 cm have generally not been performed using this technique. In cases of smaller diverticula, CP myotomy can be performed with the laser or an open procedure. For larger diverticula, a second stapler can be used. The goal is to leave less than 1 cm of common wall between the diverticula and esophagus. A report of 150 patients undergoing ESD was compared with other patients undergoing endoscopic and open techniques for the treatment of ZD. The ESD group had an average hospital stay of 0.76 days and an average time to oral intake of 0.25 days. Their mean operative time was 34 minutes. The overall complication rate was 12.7% and the major complication rate was 2%. There was one esophageal perforation, one aspiration pneumonia, and one transient vocal cord paralysis. Ninety-eight percent of patients reported improvement or complete relief of symptoms by the first postoperative visit. At a mean follow-up of 33 months, 88% of patients reported still having improved or complete relief of symptoms.[42]

Similar results were noted in 55 patients from Israel. Fifty-one of 55 patients were successfully treated with ESD while 4 patients were treated with open diverticulotomy. This was due to inadequate exposure of the common wall or an inability to safely apply the stapling device. There was a 90% symptomatic success rate with a mean follow-up period of 33 months. Patients were fed in less than 1 day and mean operative time was 22 minutes, but the average hospital stay was 2.24 days. The investigators hospitalized the patients for 1 day to detect early complications. There were 5 recurrences, which were all successfully treated with repeat ESD. Two major complications occurred, an esophageal perforation and severe esophageal edema, necessitating a feeding tube.[43]

A retrospective study of 40 patients compared the endoscopic CO_2 laser technique with ESD. Both techniques had similar improvement in dysphagia and regurgitation symptom scores, but the average length of stay was longer and the complication rate was higher in the CO_2 laser group. The increased rate of complication was attributable to 3 patients who had subcutaneous emphysema, which resolved without sequelae. Neither group developed mediastinitis, perforation, hemorrhage, recurrent laryngeal nerve injury, or death.[44]

When different open and endoscopic techniques were compared, it was reported that open procedures had a higher complication rate (11.8% vs 5.5%), higher mortality rate (1.6% vs 0.2%), longer hospital stay (7.6 vs 1.8 days), and longer time until diets were resumed (4.5 vs 1.0 days). Shorter operative times were also noted when open and endoscopic techniques were compared (mean operating room time: 83 vs 29 minutes).[42] When comparing the different endoscopic techniques, ESD was found to have a shorter hospital stay and time to oral diet compared with electrosurgery and CO_2 laser techniques. Recurrence rates were reported to be similar between the open and endoscopic techniques (5% vs 6.6%), although reported follow-up times were shorter for the endoscopic approaches. Treatment of recurrent ZD can be performed in an open manner[45] or with ESD,[46] with similar success rates (>93%). Similar to first-time treatment for ZD, open patients had higher complication rates and longer hospital stays. Despite the published advantages of the endoscopic techniques, both approaches appear to have high patient satisfaction rates, and patients would be willing to undergo either surgery again.[47]

SUMMARY

CP dysphagia and ZD can be challenging but treatable medical problems. Most patients can be diagnosed with a detailed history, modified barium swallow, or manufluorography. There is a limited role for nonsurgical interventions. Surgical intervention with open or endoscopic approaches yields similar success rates. Compared with open techniques for the treatment of ZD, endoscopic techniques have lower complication rates as well as shorter operative times, hospital stays, and time to oral intake.

REFERENCES

1. Zenker FA, von Ziemssen H. Dilatations of the esophagus. Cyclopedia of the Practice of Medicine 1878;3:46–8.
2. Watemberg S, Landau O, Avrahami R. Zenker's diverticulum: reappraisal. Am J Gastroenterol 1996;91(8):1494–8.
3. Siddiq MA, Sood S, Strachan D. Pharyngeal pouch (Zenker's diverticulum) [review]. Postgrad Med J 2001;77(910):506–11.
4. Kahrilas PJ. Upper esophageal sphincter function during antegrade and retrograde transit. Am J Med 1997;103(5A):56S–60S.
5. Veenker EA, Andersen PE, Cohen JI. Cricopharyngeal spasm and Zenker's diverticulum. Head Neck 2003;25(8):681–94.
6. Plant RL. Anatomy and physiology of swallowing in adults and geriatrics. Otolaryngol Clin North Am 1998;31(3):477–88.
7. Westrin KM, Ergün S, Carlsöö B. Zenker's diverticulum—a historical review and trends in therapy. Acta Otolaryngol 1996;116(3):351–60.
8. Fulp SR, Castell DO. Manometric aspects of Zenker's diverticulum. Hepatogastroenterology 1992;39 (2):123–6.
9. McConnel FM, Hood D, Jackson K, et al. Analysis of intrabolus forces in patients with Zenker's diverticulum. Laryngoscope 1994;104(5 Pt 1):571–81.
10. Cook IJ, Blumbergs P, Cash K, et al. Structural abnormalities of the cricopharyngeus muscle in patients with pharyngeal (Zenker's) diverticulum. J Gastroenterol Hepatol 1992;7(6):556–62.
11. Lerut T, van Raemdonck D, Guelinckx P, et al. Zenker's diverticulum: is a myotomy of the cricopharyngeus useful? How long should it be? Hepatogastroenterology 1992;39(2):127–31.
12. Zaninotto G, Costantini M, Boccù C, et al. Functional and morphological study of the cricopharyngeal muscle in patients with Zenker's diverticulum. Br J Surg 1996;83(9):1263–7.
13. Cook IJ. Oropharyngeal dysphagia. Gastroenterol Clin North Am 2009;38(3):411–3.
14. Dantas RO, Cook IJ, Dodds WJ, et al. Biomechanics of cricopharyngeal bars. Gastroenterology 1990; 99(5):1269–74.
15. Elidan J, Shochina M, Gonen B, et al. Electromyography of the inferior constrictor and cricopharyngeal muscles during swallowing. Ann Otol Rhinol Laryngol 1990;99(6 Pt 1):466–9.
16. Solt J, Bajor J, Moizs M, et al. Primary cricopharyngeal dysfunction: treatment with balloon catheter dilatation. Gastrointest Endosc 2001;54(6):767–71.
17. Zepeda-Gómez S, Montaño Loza A, Valdovinos F, et al. Endoscopic balloon catheter dilation for treatment of primary cricopharyngeal dysfunction. Dig Dis Sci 2004;49(10):1612–4.
18. Schneider I, Thumfart WF, Pototschnig C, et al. Treatment of dysfunction of the cricopharyngeal muscle with botulinum A toxin: introduction of a new, noninvasive method. Ann Otol Rhinol Laryngol 1994; 103(1):31–5.
19. Zaninotto G, Marchese Ragona R, Briani C, et al. The role of botulinum toxin injection and upper esophageal sphincter myotomy in treating oropharyngeal dysphagia. J Gastrointest Surg 2004;8(8): 997–1006.
20. Blitzer A, Brin MF. Use of botulinum toxin for diagnosis and management of cricopharyngeal achalasia. Otolaryngol Head Neck Surg 1997;116(3): 328–30.
21. Ahsan SF, Meleca RJ, Dworkin JP. Botulinum toxin injection of the cricopharyngeus muscle for the treatment of dysphagia. Otolaryngol Head Neck Surg 2000;122(5):691–5.
22. Moerman MB. Cricopharyngeal Botox injection: indications and technique. Curr Opin Otolaryngol Head Neck Surg 2006;14(6):431–6.
23. Murry T, Wasserman T, Carrau RL, et al. Injection of botulinum toxin A for the treatment of dysfunction of the upper esophageal sphincter. Am J Otolaryngol 2005;26(3):157–62.
24. Kaplan S. Paralysis of deglutition, a post-poliomyelitis complication treated by section of the cricopharyngeus muscle. Ann Surg 1951;133(4):572–3.
25. Halvorson DJ, Kuhn FA. Transmucosal cricopharyngeal myotomy with the potassium-titanyl-phosphate laser in the treatment of cricopharyngeal dysmotility. Ann Otol Rhinol Laryngol 1994;103(3):173–7.
26. Ishioka S, Sakai P, Maluf Filho F, et al. Endoscopic incision of Zenker's diverticula. Endoscopy 1995; 27:433–7.
27. Mulder CJ, den Hartog G, Robijn RJ, et al. Flexible endoscopic treatment of Zenker's diverticulum: a new approach. Endoscopy 1995;27:438–42.
28. van Overbeek JJ, Hoeksema PE, Edens ET. Microendoscopic surgery of the hypopharyngeal diverticulum using electrocoagulation or carbon dioxide laser. Ann Otol Rhinol Laryngol 1984;93: 34–6.
29. Kuhn FA, Bent JP. Zenker's diverticulotomy using the Ktp/532 laser. Laryngoscope 1992;102:946–50.
30. Dauer E, Salassa J, Iuga L, et al. Endoscopic laser vs open approach for cricopharyngeal myotomy. Otolaryngol Head Neck Surg 2006;134(5):830–5.
31. Belsey R. Functional disease of the esophagus. J Thorac Cardiovasc Surg 1966;52(2):164–88.
32. Dorion D, Brown DH, Gullane PJ. How I do it: Zenker's stapler diverticulectomy. J Otolaryngol 1994; 23(2):145–7.

33. Busaba NY, Ishoo E, Kieff D. Open Zenker's diverticulectomy using stapling techniques. Ann Otol Rhinol Laryngol 2001;110(6):498–501.

34. Bonavina L, Bona D, Abraham M, et al. Long-term results of endosurgical and open surgical approach for Zenker diverticulum. World J Gastroenterol 2007; 13(18):2586–9.

35. Mosher HP. Webs and pouches of the esophagus: their diagnosis and treatment. Surg Gynecol Obstet 1917;25:175–87.

36. Dohlman G, Mattson O. The endoscopic operation for hypopharyngeal diverticula. AMA Arch Otolaryngol 1960;71:744–52.

37. Fama AF, Moore EJ, Kasperbauer JL. Harmonic scalpel in the treatment of Zenker's diverticulum. Laryngoscope 2009;119(7):1265–9.

38. Mortensen M, Schaberg MR, Genden EM, et al. Transoral resection of short segment Zenker's diverticulum and cricopharyngeal myotomy: an alternative minimally invasive approach. Laryngoscope 2010;120(1):17–22.

39. Ho AS, Morzaria S, Damrose EJ. Carbon dioxide laser-assisted endoscopic cricopharyngeal myotomy with primary mucosal closure. Ann Otol Rhinol Laryngol 2011;120(1):33–9.

40. Collard JM, Otte JB, Kestens PJ. Endoscopic stapling technique of esophagodiverticulostomy for Zenker's diverticulum. Ann Thorac Surg 1993;56:573–6.

41. Martin-Hirsch DP, Newbegin CJ. Autosuture GIA gun: a new application in the treatment of hypopharyngeal diverticula. J Laryngol Otol 1993;107: 723–5.

42. Chang CY, Payyapilli RJ, Scher RL. Endoscopic staple diverticulostomy for Zenker's diverticulum: review of literature and experience in 159 consecutive cases. Laryngoscope 2003;113(6): 957–65.

43. Wasserzug O, Zikk D, Raziel A, et al. Endoscopically stapled diverticulostomy for Zenker's diverticulum: results of a multidisciplinary team approach. Surg Endosc 2010;24(3):637–41.

44. Miller FR, Bartley J, Otto RA. The endoscopic management of Zenker diverticulum: CO_2 laser versus endoscopic stapling. Laryngoscope 2006; 116(9):1608–11.

45. Rocco G, Deschamps C, Martel E, et al. Results of reoperation on the upper esophageal sphincter. J Thorac Cardiovasc Surg 1999;117(1):28–30 [discussion: 30–1].

46. Scher RL. Endoscopic staple diverticulostomy for recurrent Zenker's diverticulum. Laryngoscope 2003;113(1):63–7.

47. Wirth D, Kern B, Guenin MO, et al. Outcome and quality of life after open surgery versus endoscopic stapler-assisted esophagodiverticulostomy for Zenker's diverticulum. Dis Esophagus 2006;19(4):294–8.

Peroral Endoscopic Myotomy for Esophageal Achalasia: Technique, Indication, and Outcomes

Haruhiro Inoue, MD, PhD*, Kris Ma Tianle, MD, PhD,
Haruo Ikeda, MD, Toshihisa Hosoya, MD,
Manabu Onimaru, MD, PhD, Akira Yoshida, MD, PhD,
Hitomi Minami, MD, Shin-ei Kudo, MD, PhD

KEYWORDS

- Peroral endoscopic myotomy • Esophageal achalasia
- Natural orifice transluminal endoscopic surgery • POEM

The concept of natural orifice transluminal endoscopic surgery (NOTES)[1-3] has inspired endoscopists and endoscopic surgeons to create and establish a novel, less-invasive treatment even for various gastrointestinal (GI) diseases. Esophageal achalasia is a primary target of NOTES. So far, treatments, including Botox injection and pneumatic dilation, have been commonly performed as first-line endoscopic treatments for achalasia.[4,5] If those interventions are ineffective, laparoscopic myotomy is generally indicated as the next step of treatment.[6]

Peroral endoscopic myotomy (POEM) has been developed as an incisionless, minimally invasive endoscopic treatment intending a permanent cure from esophageal achalasia.[7] The concept of endoscopic myotomy was first reported around 3 decades ago,[8] but the direct incision method through the mucosal layer was not considered to be a safe and reliable approach. Pasricha and colleagues[9] recently reported the concept of tunneled submucosal myotomy using a porcine model, which enabled the closure of the mucosal-submucosal opening away from the myotomy site. Sumiyama and colleagues[10] also reported the technical usefulness of submucosal tunneling in the porcine model. Based on these experimental data, a novel method of endoscopic myotomy was developed and established by the present authors.[11]

In this article, the current techniques, applications, and clinical results of POEM are described.

INSTITUTIONAL REVIEW BOARD APPROVAL AND INFORMED CONSENT

The POEM procedure received approval from the Institutional Review Board of Showa University Northern Yokohama Hospital (approval number 0805–02, issued on August 15, 2008). Written informed consent was obtained from all patients. All patients who underwent POEM were registered in the University Hospital Medical Information Network Japan database.

INDICATIONS

All patients with achalasia can be treated by POEM. In the authors' early series, the indication for POEM was limited to the nonsigmoid-type esophagus, but the initial patient feedback to the POEM procedure was better than expected. Based on the authors' initial results, the study was opened to all grades of achalasia. More recently, the indication for POEM was further

Digestive Disease Center, Showa University Northern Yokohama Hospital, Chigasaki-Chuo 35-1, Tsuzuki-ku, Yokohama 224-8503, Japan
* Corresponding author.
E-mail address: haruinoue777@yahoo.co.jp

Thorac Surg Clin 21 (2011) 519–525
doi:10.1016/j.thorsurg.2011.08.005
1547-4127/11/$ – see front matter © 2011 Elsevier Inc. All rights reserved.

extended to the cases of failed surgical myotomy. Currently, the authors have no exceptions when considering the application of the POEM.

EQUIPMENT USED FOR POEM

A forward-viewing endoscope with an outer diameter of 9.8 mm, which is designed for routine upper GI endoscopy, is used with a transparent distal cap attachment (MH-588; Olympus, Center Valley, PA, USA [Fig. 1A]). The cap has an oblique orifice, which extends beyond the distal end of the endoscope for a distance of 1 cm and is essential for

entering and maintaining endoscopic visualization within the submucosal space. All equipment, including the endoscope itself, is sterilized using ethylene oxide gas.

A triangle-tip knife (KD-640L; Olympus) is used to dissect the submucosal layer and also to divide circular muscle bundles at the level of the esophagogastric junction (EGJ) (see Fig. 1B). The maximum diameter of the triangle-tip knife is 2.6 mm, and it will pass through the working channel of the 9.8 mm endoscope. The authors use an electrosurgical energy generator (VIO 300D, ERBE; Tübingen, Germany) that enables a spray-coagulation mode

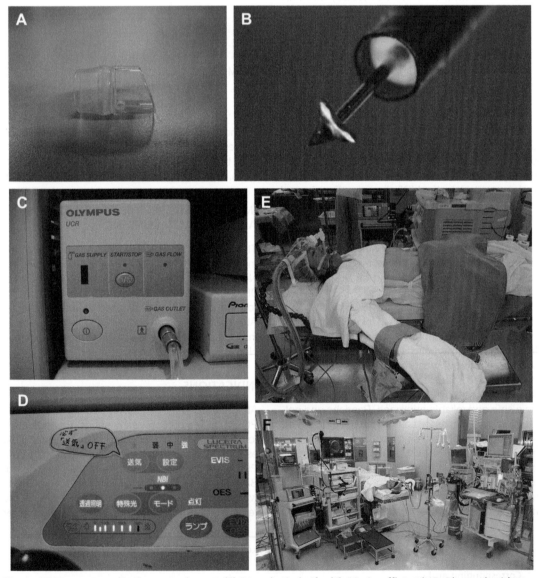

Fig. 1. (*A*) Transparent distal cap attachment. (*B*) Triangle-tip knife. (*C*) CO_2 insufflator (UC; Olympus) with standard tubing. (*D*) The standard endoscopic air pump should be turned off for the duration of the procedure. (*E, F*) The upper abdomen is prepared and then checked periodically during the procedure.

with noncontact tissue dissection. The spray-coagulation mode makes the submucosal dissection during tunnel creation much easier, faster, and with less bleeding.

A coagulating forceps (Coagrasper, FD-411QR; Olympus) is used to cauterize larger vessels when encountered during submucosal dissection.

Carbon dioxide (CO_2) gas insufflation is a critical factor to achieve a safe POEM. CO_2 delivery is provided with the aid of a CO_2 insufflator (UC; Olympus) and standard tubing (see **Fig. 1**C). Endoscopic CO_2 insufflation with a controlled gas feed of 1.2 L/min is beneficial for reducing the risk of both mediastinal emphysema and air embolization. The standard endoscopic air pump should be turned off for the duration of the procedure or air will be supplied together with CO_2 insufflation, negating any safety advantage of the CO_2 (see **Fig. 1**D).

For final closure of the mucosal entry site, hemostatic clips (EZ-CLIP, HX-110QR; Olympus) are applied. Using hemostatic clips, the mucosal entry site can be closed tightly, thereby avoiding leakage of the esophageal contents into the mediastinum.

EXAMINATIONS AND PREPARATION BEFORE POEM

Esophagram, manometry, and upper endoscopy are essential to make the correct diagnosis of esophageal achalasia. Computed tomography (CT) scan is used not only to judge the degree of esophageal dilation but also to provide information of the anatomic features of the adjacent structures.

On the day before the POEM, sennoside (2 tablets, 12 mg) is taken with liquid at bedtime. The purpose of using this laxative is to reduce the movement of the GI tract, and time of onset is 6 to 10 hours after ingestion.

Endoscopic clearance of the esophageal contents and a liquid diet is suggested, particularly for sigmoid-type achalasia on the day before the POEM. Using a large channel endoscope, esophageal contents are evacuated and cleared. Patients are fasted on the day of the POEM. During the procedure, a clear endoscopic view will be guaranteed without food and liquid residue in the esophagus. An empty esophagus also avoids aspiration during induction of anesthesia.

THE POEM PROCEDURE
Step 1: Intratracheal Intubation and CO_2 Insufflation

The procedure is performed with patients under general anesthesia. Severe mediastinal emphysema may occur if the POEM is performed with conscious sedation and without intratracheal intubation. Positive pressure ventilation reduces the risk of mediastinal emphysema. During the POEM, pneumoperitoneum occurred in 8 patients. To prevent abdominal compartment syndrome, the upper abdomen is prepared and then checked periodically during the POEM procedure (see **Fig. 1**E, F).

When the abdomen is excessively distended, drainage of the CO_2 from the abdominal cavity is performed using an injection needle.

Step 2: Creation of a Submucosal Tunnel

Mucosal entry
A submucosal injection of 10 mL of saline with 0.3% indigo carmine is performed before opening the mucosal surface (**Fig. 2**A). The point of entry usually lies on the anterior wall of the esophagus. A 2-cm longitudinal incision in the 2-o'clock position is created using dry cut mode at 50 W on effect 3 (**Fig. 3**A); this position on the esophagus leads to the lesser curvature side of the stomach without injury to the sling fibers.

A submucosal injection is generally performed at the level of the midesophagus, approximately 13 cm proximal to the gastroesophageal junction. The estimated length of the tunnel becomes 16 cm (29–45 cm).

If patients have abnormal contractions of the upper third of the esophagus, a longer myotomy is required. A long myotomy can effectively control chest pain caused by the spasm of the hypertrophied circular muscle.

Submucosal tunnel
The tunnel is created distally by using a technique similar to endoscopic submucosal dissection. The tunnel is passed over the EGJ and the gastric lumen is entered 3 cm distally. Using a triangle-tip knife (see **Fig. 1**B), the submucosal tissue is dissected using a no-touch technique with spray-coagulation mode at 50 W using effect 2. The dissection plane is located nearly on the surface of the muscularis (see **Figs. 2**B, **3**B). It is important to mention that the dissection should never be performed directly adjacent to the mucosal layer because this is the only barrier between the esophageal lumen and the mediastinum after completion of the myotomy. A mucosal opening within the distal tunnel could lead to mediastinal sepsis.

Should the submucosal dissection plane become unclear, repeated injection of saline will enhance the demarcation between the submucosal layer and muscularis propria. The width of the tunnel is about one-third of the circumference of the esophagus. The identification of the palisade

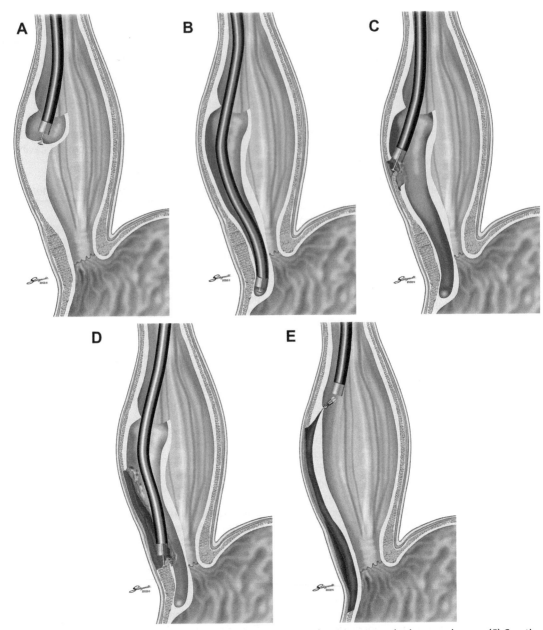

Fig. 2. Schematic depiction. (*A*) Submucosal injection and mucosal incision toward submucosal space. (*B*) Creation of submucosal tunnel. (*C*) Myotomy started at inside submucosal tunnel. (*D*) Completion of myotomy beyond esophago-gastric junction. (*E*) Closure of mucosal entry.

vessels within the submucosal layer is helpful in identifying the location of the EGJ (see **Fig. 3**C). Once the tip of the endoscope has reached the cardia, the submucosal space will be opened widely. The location of the distal margin of the tunnel can be verified using a retroflexion view from within the gastric lumen (see **Fig. 3**D). Large vessels identified within the submucosal tunnel are coagulated using hemostatic forceps in soft-coagulation mode at 80 W using effect 5.

Identification of the EGJ

A challenge with POEM concerns the identification of the EGJ from within the submucosal space. The first indicator of the location of the EGJ is the insertion depth of the endoscope from the incisors. The position of the EGJ as measured from within the lumen of the esophagus is recorded accurately before creating the submucosal tunnel. The insertion depth of the endoscope in the submucosal tunnel is similar to that of the true lumen. The

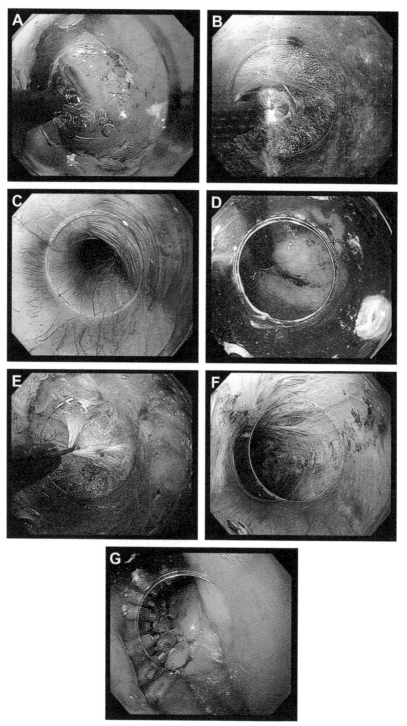

Fig. 3. (*A*) Longitudinal incision in the 2-o'clock position. (*B*) Dissection plane. (*C*) Palisade vessels within the submucosal layer. (*D*) Distal margin of the tunnel. (*E*) The sharp tip of the triangle-tip knife is used to catch circular muscle bundles and then retract them toward the esophageal lumen. (*F*) Longitudinal muscle is identified at the bottom of myotomy site. (*G*) Closure with endoscopic clips.

second indicator of the EGJ location is a marked increase in resistance when the endoscope encounters the EGJ, followed by a prompt easing when the endoscope passes through the narrowed EGJ and enters the gastric submucosal space. The third indicator of the EGJ location is the endoscopic visualization of the palisade vessels within the submucosal layer. Palisade vessels are located at the distal end of the esophagus. These vessels were identified in every case of POEM. Finally, the fourth indicator is the degree of vascularity in the submucosal layer. In the esophageal submucosal space, few vessels are observed; but when the EGJ is crossed on to the stomach, the submucosal vasculature becomes weblike and abundant.

Step 3: Endoscopic Myotomy

Dissection of the sphincter muscle
The dissection of the circular muscle bundle was initiated 2 cm distal to the mucosal entry point, more than 10 cm proximal to the EGJ (see **Fig. 2**C). The sharp tip of the triangle-tip knife is used to catch circular muscle bundles and then retract them toward the esophageal lumen (see **Fig. 3**E). The circular fibers are divided using a spray-coagulation current at 50 W using effect 2. Only circular muscle bundles should be lifted and then cut by electrocautery. A plane of longitudinal muscle is identified at the bottom of the myotomy site (see **Fig. 3**F). This intramuscular space is the ideal space to be continuously dissected while maintaining the longitudinal muscle layer intact. By attempting to keep the longitudinal muscle layer intact, the endoscopist can potentially reduce the risk of injury to the mediastinal structures surrounding the esophagus.

The division of the sphincter muscle is continued from the proximal side of the EGJ toward the stomach until the endoscope passes through the narrowed segment at the level of the collar-sling fibers. The myotomy is extended for a distance of 2 cm on to the stomach (see **Fig. 2**D). Easy passage of the endoscope through the EGJ without resistance from within the native lumen provides confirmation of complete myotomy.

Avoiding gastroesophageal reflux disease
In laparoscopic myotomy, a partial antireflux procedure, such as Dr Dor fundoplication, is routinely performed to prevent postoperative gastroesophageal reflux disease (GERD) because adjacent structures surrounding the distal esophagus are inevitably dissected. With POEM, no antireflux procedure is performed because the endoscopist never touches the phrenoesophageal membrane, which surrounds the abdominal esophagus and

top of the cardia. Theoretically, the hiatal attachments are left untouched and the flap-valve mechanism intact.

To reduce the risk of post-POEM GERD, anterior myotomy in the 2-o'clock position on the circumference of the esophagus (patients positioned supine) directs the myotomy to the lesser gastric curvature without disturbing the acute angle of His, which is located the 8-o'clock position.

Myotomy length and myotomy direction
A major advantage of POEM is the ability to tailor myotomy length. Myotomy length is routinely greater than 10 cm. In patients with chest pain caused by the abnormal contractions of hypertrophied muscle within the esophageal body, a long myotomy is made and all abnormal contractions (endoscopically visible and measured with manometry) are incorporated into the site of circular muscle division. In the authors' series, the longest myotomy was 25 cm in 2 cases of vigorous achalasia.

We can also easily control myotomy direction. In the surgically failed case, POEM is placed on the posterior esophageal wall to avoid previous surgical site scarring.

Step 4: Closure of Mucosal Entry

Before closure of the mucosal entry site, 20 mL of saline with 80 mg gentamycin is sprayed into the submucosal tunnel. The mucosal entry site, usually 2 to 3 cm long, is closed with 5 to 10 endoscopic clips (see **Figs. 2**E and **3**G). Even when mucosal entry is elongated to a location over the myotomy site, tight mucosal closure with clips avoids leakage of the esophageal contents into the mediastinum. The successful closure of mucosal entry is confirmed by the endoscopic appearance. At the completion of the procedure, the endoscope was again inserted into the native lumen and down to the stomach to confirm smooth passage through the EGJ.

Postoperative Care

Gastroscopy
The aim is to confirm mucosal integrity. If no mucosal damage is found, a liquid meal is started and then gradually advanced; if a mucosal defect is present, the patients are fasted until confirmation of defect closure. Fortunately in the authors' series, they had no experience of mucosal damage. It should be reinforced that after complete myotomy, the mucosa layer is an only barrier between the esophageal lumen and mediastinum.

Contrast media swallow
An esophagram is also important to confirm the smooth passage of contrast media through the

EGJ without leakage or stasis. Adequate esophageal emptying and the absence of leak enables oral intake to resume. Patients begin by drinking liquid on day 1, a soft diet on postoperative day 2, and a normal diet on postoperative day 3 following the POEM.

Antibiotics

An intravenous infusion of antibiotics is delivered for 3 days after the POEM, and then patients are transitioned to an additional 4 days of oral antibiotics.

CLINICAL RESULTS

The first case was performed on September 8, 2008. One hundred five consecutive patients, including 16 patients with sigmoid achalasia, received POEM. In all patients, the dysphagia score recovered dramatically except for 1. In most of the patients, chest pain reduced or totally disappeared. No major complications occurred, such as mediastinitis, hemorrhage, or mucosal necrosis. One patient developed peritonitis, which was controlled nonoperatively with antibiotics and observation. Long myotomy was performed in most patients without any cases of mediastinitis. This finding suggests that the tight closure of the mucosal entry site using the endoscopic clipping avoids the development of a leak. Even though the CT scan detected pneumomediastinum in several patients after POEM, there were no clinical sequelae related to this finding. In 1 patient, a chest tube was placed to control pneumothorax. In this particular case air was insufflated instead of CO_2 gas. No patients received additional therapy for achalasia, except 1 patient who received a single 20 mm pneumatic dilation. Eighteen patients developed endoscopic evidence of gastroesophageal reflux. Six of 18 patients developed symptoms of GERD, and all responded to therapy with proton pump inhibitors.

In this series, there were 7 patients with failure of a prior surgical myotomy that was successfully treated by POEM. The symptom score was dramatically improved in those patients.

SUMMARY

POEM is a novel incisionless treatment of esophageal achalasia. POEM can be applied to any grade of achalasia, and short-term results are excellent.

REFERENCES

1. Kalloo AN, Singh VK, Jagannath SB, et al. Flexible transgastric peritoneoscopy: a novel approach to diagnostic and therapeutic interventions. Gastrointest Endosc 2004;60:114–7.
2. Zorron R, Filgueiras M, Maggioni LC, et al. NOTES. Transvaginal cholecystectomy: report of the first case. Surg Innov 2007;14:279–83.
3. Marescaux J, Dallemagne B, Perretta S, et al. Surgery without scars: report of transluminal cholecystectomy in a human being. Arch Surg 2007; 142:823–6.
4. Spiess AE, Kahrilas PJ. Treating achalasia: from whalebone to laparoscope. JAMA 1998;280:638.
5. Pehlivanov N, Pasricha PJ. Achalasia: Botox, dilation or laparoscopic surgery in 2006. Neurogastroenterol Motil 2006;18:799–804.
6. Woltman TA, Pellegrini CA, Oelschlager BK. Achalasia. Surg Clin North Am 2005;85:483–93.
7. Inoue H, Minami H, Satodate H, et al. First clinical experience of submucosal endoscopic myotomy for esophageal achalasia with no skin incision. Gastrointest Endosc 2009;69:AB122.
8. Ortega JA, Madureri V, Perez I. Endoscopic myotomy in the treatment of achalasia. Gastrointest Endosc 1980;26:8–10.
9. Pasricha PJ, Hawari R, Ahmed I, et al. Submucosal endoscopic esophageal myotomy: a novel experimental approach for the treatment of achalasia. Endoscopy 2007;39:761–4.
10. Sumiyama K, Gostout CJ, Rajan E, et al. Submucosal endoscopy with mucosal flap safety valve. Gastrointest Endosc 2007;65:688–94.
11. Inoue H, Minami H, Kobayash Y, et al. Per-oral endoscopic myotomy (POEM) for esophageal achalasia. Endoscopy 2010;42:265–71.

Esophageal Preservation in Esophageal High-Grade Dysplasia and Intramucosal Adenocarcinoma

Toshitaka Hoppo, MD, PhD*, Shah D. Rachit, MD,
Blair A. Jobe, MD

KEYWORDS

• Esophageal preservation • High-grade dysplasia
• Intramucosal adenocarcinoma • Endoscopic therapy

In the last 30 years, the incidence of esophageal cancer, especially adenocarcinoma, has been rapidly increasing in the United States[1,2] and it now accounts for approximately 70% of all esophageal cancers in Western countries.[3,4] Barrett esophagus (BE) is a well-known risk factor for esophageal adenocarcinoma, and progression of metaplasia through dysplasia to adenocarcinoma is a widely accepted theory of esophageal carcinogenesis. High-grade dysplasia (HGD) has a high rate of progression to cancer, and the rate of synchronous cancer in the surgically resected specimens of patients with a preoperative diagnosis of only HGD has been reported to be approximately 40%.[5,6] Based on this, esophagectomy has been recommended as the standard of care to treat HGD. However, esophagectomy is associated with high mortality and morbidity even in experienced centers.[7,8] Lymph node metastasis is unlikely (<2%) in patients with HGD and intramucosal (T1a) adenocarcinoma.[9–11]

As the guidelines put forth by the Society of Thoracic Surgeons state, the management of HGD and intramucosal adenocarcinoma remains controversial.[12] With the widespread acceptance of BE surveillance programs, the number of patients with HGD and/or intramucosal adenocarcinoma has increased,[13,14] and interest in the treatment strategies for esophageal preservation has grown. Esophageal preservation indicates any endoluminal procedure that is used in an attempt to completely eradicate disease, while preserving the anatomic structure of the esophagus. With the recent advances in both technology and technique, the concept of esophageal preservation has become a reality and this approach has changed the current management of HGD and intramucosal adenocarcinoma. However, the risk of lymph node metastasis increases from 2% to 25% when a tumor invades into the submucosal layer, and the presence of lymph node metastasis significantly decreases chances for long-term survival.[15,16] Therefore, it is essential to select patients who are appropriate for esophagus-preserving approaches, such as mucosal ablation and endoscopic resection, based on pretreatment clinical staging. This article describes the status of currently available esophagus-preserving options and discusses the strategy for treating HGD and intramucosal adenocarcinoma.

PATIENT SELECTION

For the esophagus-preserving approaches, patient selection is a critical component of pretreatment work-up. Therefore, the pretreatment

Division of Thoracic and Foregut Surgery, Department of Cardiothoracic Surgery, University of Pittsburgh Medical Center, 5200 Centre Avenue, Suite 715, Pittsburgh, PA 15232, USA
* Corresponding author.
E-mail address: hoppot2@upmc.edu

Thorac Surg Clin 21 (2011) 527–540
doi:10.1016/j.thorsurg.2011.08.009
1547-4127/11/$ – see front matter © 2011 Elsevier Inc. All rights reserved.

work-up should include accurate, meticulous endoscopic examination with extensive biopsies and the assessment for lymph node involvement and metastatic disease using endoscopic ultrasonography (EUS), endoscopic resection for staging, and positron emission tomography (PET)/computed tomography (CT).

It is important to identify patients at high risk for progressing to cancer or for harboring synchronous invasive cancer with possible lymph node metastasis. All risk factors based on the endoscopic findings and histologic characteristics are summarized in **Table 1**. Patients with multifocal HGD have a high risk of concomitant invasive cancer in the range of 60% to 78%.[13,17] In contrast, patients with unifocal (ie, limited or focal), flat (no nodularity) HGD are less likely to have concomitant cancer[13,14] or to progress to cancer.[17,18] Furthermore, histologic characteristics such as squamous-type histology, lymphovascular invasion, poor differentiation, and a nodule size greater than 3 cm likely increase the risk of lymphatic spread.[19–22] Long-segment BE may be associated with sampling error, and even short-segment BE may represent a similar cancer risk as long-segment disease.[23]

DETECTION OF DYSPLASIA/CANCER

1. *Biopsy.* Although the Seattle Protocol (biopsies with jumbo forceps in 4 quadrants, along every centimeter of endoscopically apparent disease, with additional biopsies taken from suspicious areas) has been widely accepted, only 2% of the esophageal surface area at a given level can be obtained using 4-quadrant biopsies, and most lesions may be missed. Furthermore, significant interobserver variability exists among pathologists in determining dysplasia[24] despite histologic criteria for dysplasia being accepted nearly 20 years ago.[25] Although 2 experienced pathologists have been encouraged to confirm histology, histologic examination alone may be inadequate to make an accurate diagnosis and evaluate the extent of disease. Therefore, alternative methods including flow cytometry,[26,27] loss of heterozygosity,[28] immunohistochemistry (in particular for p53),[28] and computerized morphometry[29] have been investigated with some encouraging results.

2. *Novel imaging technology.* The management of HGD and intramucosal adenocarcinoma starts with an appropriate endoscopic examination by an experienced endoscopist. The high quality of endoscopic images is crucial to detect subtle esophageal mucosal abnormalities, which may harbor neoplasia. Dysplasia and even intramucosal adenocarcinoma cannot be distinguished from nondysplastic BE using conventional white light endoscopy. Since the introduction of high-resolution endoscopy using high-quality charge-coupled devices (CCDs), many novel imaging techniques and devices have been introduced, potentially leading to the targeted biopsy. The ideal imaging technique would have the following characteristics: high sensitivity with low false-positive rate for dysplasia, the ability to scan a wide area with microscopic resolution in real time, the ability to differentiate dysplasia from inflammation-related changes, high interobserver agreement, ability to localize dysplastic areas for targeted biopsy, and low cost. At present, no

---

Table 1
Risk factors for esophageal preservation

Concurrent Cancer or Progression to Invasive Cancer	
Low Risk	**High Risk**
Unifocal (limited or focal), flat HGD	Multifocal HGD, HGD with nodules
Lymph Node Involvement	
Low Risk	**High Risk**
Type I, IIa <20 mm, IIb, IIc <10 mm	Type I, II >30 mm, type III
Well or moderately differentiated adenocarcinoma (grading G1/G2)	Poorly differentiated adenocarcinoma (grading G3), squamous cell carcinoma
Lesions limited to the mucosa	Invasion into submucosal layer
No lymphovascular invasion	Presence of lymphovascular invasion

Type I, polypoid type; II, flat type; IIa, flat, elevated; IIb, level with the mucosa; IIc, slightly depressed; III, ulcerated type.
  Data from Hoppo T, Jobe BA. Esophageal preservation in the setting of esophageal high-grade dysplasia and superficial cancer. Ann Gastroenterol Hepatol 2011, in press; and Japanese Gastric Cancer Association. Japanese classification of gastric carcinoma - 2nd English edition. Gastric Cancer 1998;1(1):10–24.

single imaging modality exhibits all of these characteristics, and neither of the new diagnostic modalities has yet become routine practice.

Magnified Endoscopy

High-resolution endoscopy and magnified endoscopy have significantly increased the sensitivity and specificity in differentiating mucosal lesions.[30] High-resolution endoscopes are capable of discriminating objects that are as small as 0.01 mm. Magnified endoscopy can produce an increase in image size of up to 150-fold. These technologies are often used with additional enhancement techniques such as chromoendoscopy and narrow band imaging[31] to facilitate the detection of subtle mucosal abnormalities and direct clinicians to the targeted biopsy.

Chromoendoscopy

Chromoendoscopy is a method for enhancing tissue characterization, differentiation, or diagnosis by the topical application of contrast agents (dyes) such as methylene blue and indigo carmine during endoscopic examination.[32] Approximately 90% of dysplastic tissues can be highlighted as either an unstained or more lightly stained area[33]; however, the results of methylene-blue–directed biopsies have been conflicting.[34,35] Acetic acid (vinegar) is not a coloring agent, but acetic acid can highlight the surface structure of epithelium by interacting with the glycoprotein layer that covers the mucosa and breaking disulphide bonds. As a result, Barrett and gastric columnar epithelium can be identified as a reddish area, whereas the normal squamous epithelium remains whitish.[36] A recent prospective study showed high reliability of vinegar staining to identify specialized columnar epithelium with high accuracy (90%), sensitivity (100%), and specificity (82%).[37] A staining interpretation is examiner dependent and chromoendoscopy is associated with interobserver variability.

Narrow Band Imaging

Narrow band imaging (NBI) is an optical filter technology that uses narrowed bandwidths of blue (440–460 nm) and green (540–560 nm) light waves to enhance the superficial capillaries and mucosal structures by optimizing the absorbance and scattering characteristics of light.[34] NBI is usually used in combination with advanced endoscopy such as high-resolution endoscopy. A recent meta-analysis showed high sensitivity (96%) and specificity (94%) in discriminating HGD in a field of BE.[35] Furthermore, a prospective, blinded, tandem endoscopy study showed that high-resolution endoscopy with NBI can detect more patients with dysplasia

and higher grades of dysplasia with fewer biopsies compared with standard-resolution endoscopy.[38]

Confocal Laser Endomicroscopy

Confocal laser endomicroscopy (CLE) is a new technology for examining the mucosal histology in real time in vivo during an endoscopic procedure. A microscope that can magnify the mucosa 1000 times is built in the tip of standard endoscope, and microscopic imaging of cells can then be obtained. Based on the difference in the microscopic structures of epithelial cells (ie, columnar cells, squamous cells), normal esophageal cells can be distinguished from intestinal metaplasia, dysplasia, and cancer (**Fig. 1**).[39,40] Following the intravenous injection of a contrast agent, a probe is introduced through the endoscopic working channel and a low-power laser is applied to the mucosa. CLE provides in vivo assessment of mucosal histopathologic characteristics in real time by detecting the fluorescent light coming back from the tissue.[41] CLE has shown high accuracy and interobserver agreement in the detection of neoplasia in BE.[42,43] The recent international, prospective, multicenter, randomized controlled study involving 97 patients with BE showed a significant increase in sensitivity, from 45% to 76%, and a reduction in biopsies in 39% of patients when CLE was used in combination with white light endoscopy or NBI, or both.[44] Because only a small area of mucosa is examined using CLE, CLE should be used in combination with other modalities to screen and identify the suspicious area before CLE.

Autofluorescence Imaging

Autofluorescence imaging (AFI) uses the laser light used during the endoscopic procedure to stimulate the natural fluorescence of the esophageal mucosa. Each tissue emits a specific wavelength of light in the visible spectrum. The fluorescence is then captured and processed by a computer, showing the difference between normal and abnormal mucosa, which is seen in real time during the endoscopic procedure. A recent multicenter, randomized trial showed that an AFI-guided approach improved the diagnostic yield for neoplasia compared with the conventional approach with 4-quadrant biopsies.[45] However, its clinical usefulness has been limited because of its poor image quality and high false-positive rates. To minimize false-positive rates, endoscopic trimodal imaging (AFI combined with high-resolution endoscopy and NBI) has been investigated. The latest multicenter, randomized controlled trial involving 87 patients with BE showed that trimodal imaging significantly improves the detection of HGD and intramucosal cancer

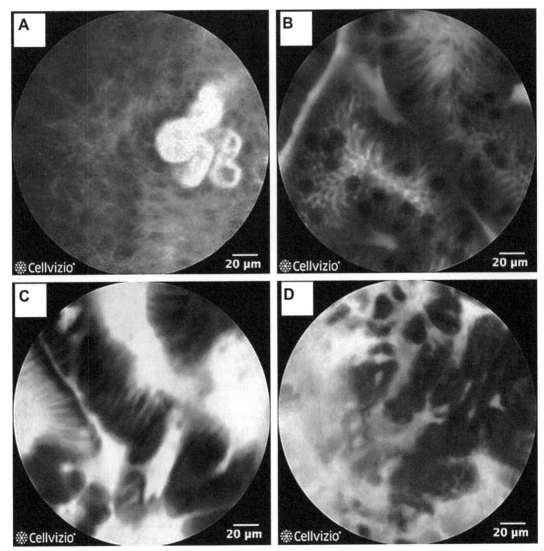

Fig. 1. CLE. (*A*) Normal squamous epithelium shows square-shaped cells. (*B*) BE shows uniform columnar-lined epithelium with mucin-containing goblet cells (*black round structure*). (*C*) High-grade dysplasia shows completely disorganized epithelium. (*D*) Adenocarcinoma shows abrupt changes to so-called black cells. (*Reproduced from Mauna Kea Technologies, Inc; with permission.*)

compared with standard endoscopy, and NBI reduced the false-positive rate of high-resolution endoscopy plus AFI from 71% to 48%; however, the addition of NBI has limited value, and trimodal imaging cannot replace the standard 4-quadrant biopsy protocol at present.[39]

ASSESSMENT OF CLINICAL STAGING

The purpose of clinical staging is to exclude submucosal involvement (T1b) and any possibility of lymph node involvement and metastatic disease, any of which would make the esophagus-preserving approaches inappropriate.

EUS

EUS has been an important component in the clinical staging of patients with HGD and intramucosal adenocarcinoma. Although a recent meta-analysis showed that the pooled sensitivity and specificity for diagnosing T1 stage cancer were 81.6% and 99.4%, respectively,[40] EUS cannot discriminate accurately between T1a and T1b esophageal tumors with the current technology. Furthermore, a recent retrospective study showed that even high-frequency miniprobe (20 or 30 MHz) still has limitations in overall accuracy (73.5%), sensitivity (62%), and specificity (76.5%) for discriminating between T1a and T1b tumors.[46] In addition, EUS is not an effective tool to detect HGD or cancer within a field of BE.[47] In HGD and intramucosal adenocarcinoma, the major role of EUS is to exclude lymph node metastasis.

PET/CT

CT has been shown to be less accurate than EUS in determining nodal staging in esophageal cancer, whereas EUS is ineffective in the detection of metastatic disease. Therefore, both modalities should be performed for the clinical staging. Previous studies showed that approximately 25% of patients with esophageal cancer have metastatic disease identified by fluorodeoxyglucose (FDG)-PET, and this yield of PET/CT is far superior to the combination of EUS and CT scan.[48,49] In HGD and intramucosal adenocarcinoma, the major role of PET/CT is to exclude metastatic disease.

Endoscopic Mucosal Resection for Staging

Because EUS may not be sufficiently reliable to exclude submucosal invasion in early esophageal cancer, endoscopic mucosal resection (EMR) is essential to determine the accurate clinical staging if a nodule is identified. EMR provides specimens including both mucosa and submucosa, allowing the histologic assessment of lateral and deep margins. Therefore, EMR can reliably determine the T stage of intramucosal esophageal lesions (ie, differentiating T1a from T1b). A positive lateral margin can be addressed with further endoscopic intervention, but a positive deep margin should be considered for esophagectomy.

For staging purposes, the mucosal and submucosal layers have been subdivided into thirds, with each third going deeper into the esophageal wall, such that T1 tumors now have 6 different layers of invasion: $T1m_1$ to $T1m_3$ (m_1 = limited to the epithelial layer; m_2 = invades lamina propria; m_3 = invades into, but not through, muscularis mucosae) and $T1sm_1$ to $T1sm_3$ (different thirds of the submucosa). A recent review involving the pooled outcomes of 7645 patients with submucosal (T1b) esophageal cancer showed that the rate of lymph node involvement is significantly increased from $T1sm_1$ to $T1sm_3$ (6%, 23%, and 58%, respectively).[50] Highly selected patients with $T1sm_1$ tumor could be candidates for esophagus-preserving approaches, although further study is required.

ESOPHAGUS-PRESERVING ENDOLUMINAL APPROACHES

Esophagus-preserving endoluminal approaches include mucosal ablation and endoscopic resection.

Both approaches attempt to destroy or remove the abnormal esophageal epithelium, which is then replaced by normal neosquamous lining, likely with normalization of the molecular baseline and a reset of the cancer risk, when tissue healing occurs in a nonacidic environment.[51] Therefore, strict acid suppression with high-dose proton pump inhibitor (PPI) and nocturnal H_2 blockade is an essential component of postprocedure management.

Mucosal Ablation

Ablation therapies include photodynamic therapy, radiofrequency ablation (RFA), and cryotherapy. Of these ablation therapies, photodynamic therapy has been abandoned because of serious complications such as stricture formation and photosensitivity. Photodynamic therapy is currently performed for palliative purposes to treat obstructing dysphagia in advanced disease.[52] Mucosal ablation therapies often require several applications and this should be discussed with the patient before the initiation of treatment. The common drawback of ablation therapy is that there is no specimen available for histopathologic examination.

RFA
RFA using the HALO system (BarrX Medical Inc, Sunnyvale, CA) is the most commonly used ablation therapy. This system includes either an ablation balloon catheter (HALO[360]) for circumferential ablation or an endoscope-mounted device (HALO[90]) for more focal ablation to deliver a high-power, ultrashort burst of ablative energy to the abnormal esophageal epithelium (**Fig. 2**). The energy delivered provides uniform treatment to a depth of about 500 µm. The depth of treatment is therefore limited to the mucosal layer and the risk of stricture formation is significantly reduced. Because of the limited depth of treatment, RFA is not indicated for the treatment of invasive cancer. The multicenter, randomized, sham-controlled trial involving 127 patients with dysplastic BE showed that 81% of patients with HGD had complete eradication of dysplasia with RFA, compared with 19% in the control group (no RFA) ($P<.001$), and patients who underwent RFA had significantly less disease progression and fewer cancers during the follow-up of 12 months.[53] The rate of stricture formation was 6%. A recent follow-up study of this trial showed that patients' quality of life significantly improved after the RFA treatment, although most patients were worried about esophageal cancer and esophagectomy before the RFA treatment.[54]

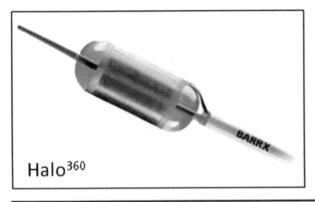

Halo³⁶⁰

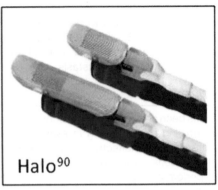

Halo⁹⁰

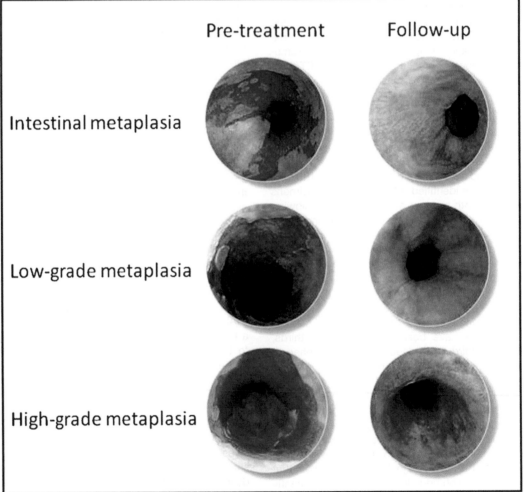

Fig. 2. RFA therapy. The upper panels show the balloon-based system Halo³⁶⁰ (*left*) and the endoscope-mounted system Halo⁹⁰ (*right*). The lower panel shows the endoscopic of pretreatment findings and the findings at follow-up for intestinal metaplasia (*top*), low-grade dysplasia (*middle*), and high-grade dysplasia (*bottom*). (*Reproduced from* BARRX Medical, Inc; with permission. The use of any BARRX photo or image does not imply BARRX review or endorsement of any article or publication.)

Cryotherapy

Cryotherapy is the latest ablation technique, involving the topical application of aerosolized liquid nitrogen or carbon dioxide onto the abnormal esophageal epithelium. This application causes intracellular disruption and ischemia but preserves the extracellular matrix and thereby promotes less fibrosis. A venting system such as a nasogastric tube is required to help excessive nitrogen gas escape from the esophagus and stomach, thus preventing perforation of the gastrointestinal tract. In a prospective open-label study involving 31 nonoperative candidates with either HGD or intramucosal carcinoma, elimination of cancer or downstaging of HGD was achieved in 68% of patients with HGD and 80% with intramucosal carcinoma during a median follow-up of 12 months.[55] A recent retrospective study involving 98 patients with HGD showed that 97% had complete eradication of HGD with no esophageal perforation.[56] Despite these encouraging results, cryotherapy has not met with widespread acceptance because of its nonuniform application using a handheld catheter, the fogging of the scope lens, risk of perforation, and the prolonged duration of the therapy.

Endoscopic Resection

Cure of HGD and intramucosal adenocarcinoma can be accomplished by removal of the segment of abnormal esophageal epithelium. The major complication is stricture formation, especially when more than 75% of the esophageal mucosal circumference is resected in a single setting,[57] with small series reporting stricture rates of 70% to 80% with circumferential EMR.[58,59]

EMR

Currently, EMR is commonly used as both a diagnostic and a therapeutic tool. The endoscopic cap resection technique and the ligate-and-cut technique are the most commonly used methods of EMR. A randomized trial to compare these 2 techniques has shown similar efficacy.[60] Both methods start with the injection of normal saline into the submucosal space to lift the lesions away from the muscularis propria, and the mucosal-submucosal complex is then suctioned into a cap mounted on an endoscope, thus creating a pseudopolyp. The pseudopolyp is then resected by being captured at its base with a cautery snare. The specimen is retrieved, pinned to a piece of cork, and placed into preservative solution before processing for histologic examination. A novel multiband mucosectomy device (Duette, Cook Medical Inc., Bloomington, IN, USA) has been introduced and is commonly used in practice. Ligation and subsequent resection can be performed immediately without removal of the endoscope by passing a polypectomy snare through the ligator handle. EMR is indicated for tumors less than or equal to 2 cm in diameter. Piecemeal excision of larger lesions (>2 cm) is acceptable but is associated with incomplete resection and compromised histologic assessment, likely leading to the development of metachronous lesions.

In an early, single-institution, retrospective report involving 115 patients with HGD and intramucosal adenocarcinoma, 98% of patients achieved complete response to EMR. However, during a mean follow-up of 34 months, 30% of patients developed metachronous cancers.[61] The risk factors most frequently associated with recurrence after endoscopic resection include piecemeal resection, long-segment BE, no ablative therapy for BE after a complete response, multifocal neoplasia, and time until complete response greater than 10 months (**Box 1**).[62] Patients therefore need to understand that intensive surveillance is required after endoscopic resection and that the risk for metachronous lesions is present. To prevent recurrences, focal EMR to resect nodules followed by RFA to treat any residual flat Barrett epithelium has been investigated. A recent multicenter, prospective study of this combination therapy, involving 24 patients with HGD or intramucosal adenocarcinoma, showed that neoplasia was eradicated in 95% of patients and no neoplasia recurred during a median follow-up of 22 months.[63] Because RFA does not cause significant scarring of the esophageal wall, EMR can be used as an escape treatment after RFA.

Endoscopic submucosal dissection

Endoscopic submucosal dissection (ESD) is an advanced endoscopic resection technique for en bloc removal of lesions larger than 2 cm in diameter, thus providing more accurate histologic assessment for the lateral and deep margins of lesions, with the expectation of preventing the development of metachronous lesions. ESD starts with marking around the lesions using electrocautery. After the marking, the lesion is lifted away from the muscularis propria by injecting a solution such as sodium hyaluronate into the submucosal space. Sodium hyaluronate can stay longer in the

---

Box 1
Risk factors potentially associated with recurrence after endoscopic resection of early esophageal cancer

1. Piecemeal resection

2. Long-segment BE

3. No ablative therapy for BE after complete response

4. Time until complete response >10 months

5. Multifocal neoplasia

submucosal space than normal saline or glycerol, and may be better suitable for ESD. Mucosal cutting is then performed to create the entry to the submucosal space by using a specialized endoscopic electrocautery needle knife. Once access to the submucosal layer is achieved, tension and countertension are maintained by an endoscope-mounted cap that is placed in the plane between the mucosal-submucosal complex and the muscularis propria. The needle knife is then deployed via the endoscopic working channel, and the attachments and bridging vessels between these 2 layers are dissected. At the completion of this procedure, the tumor can be resected en bloc regardless of its size (**Fig. 3**).[64]

Although no randomized controlled study to compare ESD with EMR has been performed, ESD may be superior to EMR because of the availability of en bloc specimen. Because ESD has not been so often applied for the treatment of HGD and intramucosal adenocarcinoma, there are insufficient data to show the efficacy of ESD in this setting. A Japanese group reported the long-term outcomes of 84 patients who underwent ESD to treat superficial esophageal squamous cell cancer.[65] En bloc resection and complete resection were achieved in 100% and 88% of patients, respectively, and the 5-year cause-specific survival of patients with intramucosal lesions was 100%. Major complications such as perforation occurred in 4% of patients, and 18% developed benign esophageal stricture requiring dilation. This study clearly suggests that ESD could be a curative treatment option for HGD and intramucosal adenocarcinoma. However, ESD for BE may be technically more complicated than ESD for gastric cancer or esophageal squamous cell cancer because of its location in the distal esophagus, close to the gastroesophageal junction, and the submucosal scarring caused by reflux-induced inflammation.

Transoral endoscopic inner-layer esophagectomy

All endoscopic approaches are currently associated with compromised histologic assessment, sampling error, and the requirement of subsequent interventions and life-long surveillance. To overcome these limitations, we have shown the feasibility of transoral endoscopic inner-layer esophagectomy (TEE) as a possible 1-step diagnostic and therapeutic approach in the preclinical setting.[66] The procedure involves a circumferential, long-sleeve resection of the entire abnormal

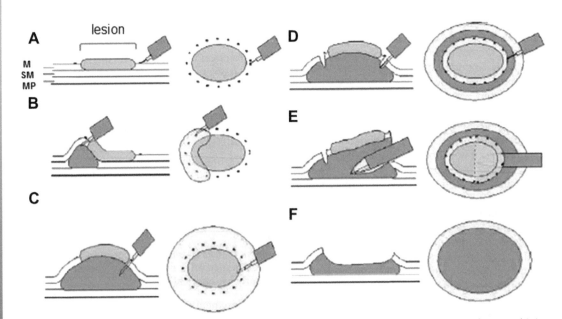

Fig. 3. The technique of ESD. (*A*) Placement of markings around the lesion to be resected. (*B*) Submucosal injection of sodium hyaluronate. (*C*) Mucosal elevation with submucosal injection under and around the lesion. (*D*) Mucosal incision around the tumor. (*E*) Submucosal dissection using a needle knife through a cap attached to the tip of the endoscope. (*F*) En-bloc resection of the lesion. M, mucosa; MP, muscularis propria; SM, submucosa. (*Reproduced from* Yamamoto H, Kawata H, Sunada K, et al. Successful en-bloc resection of large superficial tumors in the stomach and colon using sodium hyaluronate and small-caliber-tip transparent hood. Endoscopy 2003;35(8):691; with permission.)

esophageal lining using endoscopy. A small-diameter plastic cable is brought retrograde through a gastrostomy and attached to a proximal cuff of mucosal-submucosal complex. By drawing back on the plastic cable, the entire mucosal-submucosal complex is stripped away from the muscularis propria similarly to the open inversion technique described by Akiyama[67] **(Fig. 4)**. However, the major concern after circumferential mucosal resection is severe stricture formation.

Biologic scaffold materials composed of xenogeneic extracellular matrix (ECM) have been investigated extensively in regenerative medicine for their ability to modify the default tissue healing response in the esophagus.[68–70] ECM has been shown to remodel the default tissue via neoepithelialization rather than scar formation[68,69] and to successfully prevent a stricture formation after aggressive, circumferential endoscopic resection.[70] In this context, we successfully performed TEE followed by ECM placement in 5 patients with HGD and intramucosal adenocarcinoma.[71] All patients underwent a long, circumferential mucosal resection, and developed mild segmental strictures that were, in most cases, easily dilated **(Fig. 5)**. Except for 1 patient, none have had clinically significant dysphagia, and no recurrence of cancer has been observed on short-term follow-up. ECM potentially enables a more aggressive and en bloc endoscopic resection.

LONG-TERM OUTCOMES OF ESOPHAGUS-PRESERVING APPROACHES

Knowledge of the long-term outcomes of patients who have undergone esophagus-preserving approaches is limited. In a single, large, prospective study involving 349 patients with HGD and intramucosal adenocarcinoma who underwent esophagus-preserving approaches such as ablation therapy and endoscopic resection,[62] 96.6% of patients achieved complete response and only 3.7% required surgery during a mean follow-up of 5 years. None of the patients died of adenocarcinoma. Furthermore, in patients who received ablation therapy for persistent or recurrent BE, 16.5% developed a metachronous neoplasia during follow-up, compared with 28.3% in the group that did not receive ablation therapy. These results suggest that additional ablation therapy for BE is effective in reducing the development of metachronous neoplasia, and esophagus-preserving approaches in this setting are durable.

MANAGEMENT AFTER ESOPHAGUS-PRESERVING APPROACHES

Successful endoscopic therapies are highly dependent on rigorous follow-up and strict acid suppression with high-dose PPI and nocturnal H_2 blockade after the intervention. Because BE is caused by gastroesophageal reflux disease, a surgical repair of gastroesophageal reflux disease

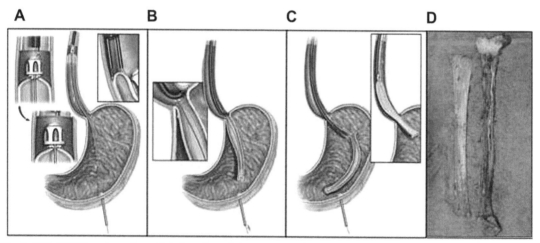

Fig. 4. TEE. (*A*) After circumferential elevation of the mucosa-submucosa complex (MSC), a vein stripper is secured to the proximal cuff of the MSC. By drawing back on the vein stripper, the MSC sleeve is inverted to facilitate submucosal dissection and stripping. (*B*) The diseased part of the MSC is dissected away from the muscularis propria and inverted into the stomach. (*C*) Before oral retrieval of resected MSC, the sleeve of the MSC is placed outside-in by drawing the trailing suture cranially. (*D*) The resection length of the MSC was evaluated macroscopically by comparing with the corresponding muscularis propria tube in a swine model. (*Reproduced from* Witteman B, Foxwell TJ, Monsheimer S, et al. Transoral endoscopic inner-layer esophagectomy: management of high-grade dysplasia and superficial cancer with organ preservation. J Gastrointest Surg 2009;13(12):2106–8; with permission.)

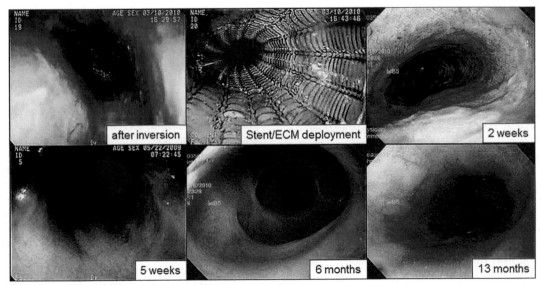

Fig. 5. The representative endoscopic views of each stage in the procedure and follow-up. (*Upper row*) Left panel: 8-cm-long circumferential muscularis propria was exposed after resection of the sleeve of the MSC. Middle panel: a stent was deployed, resulting in the gentle compression of the ECM against the muscularis propria. Right panel: immediately following stent removal at 2-weeks follow-up. The ECM was incorporated into the area of resection. (*Bottom row*) Left panel: at 5-weeks after surgery, the ECM was no longer visible and the resected region was entirely covered by squamous epithelium. Middle panel: at 6-months follow-up. The esophageal mucosa appeared normal with short-segment circumferential stricture formation. Pneumatic dilation was performed. Right panel: at 13-months follow-up. The resected region was covered with normal-appearing squamous epithelium and minimal narrowing. (*Reproduced from* Badylak SF, Hoppo T, Nieponice A, et al. Esophageal preservation in five male patients after endoscopic inner-layer circumferential resection in the setting of superficial cancer: a regenerative medicine approach with a biologic scaffold. Tissue Eng Part A 2011;17(11–12):1646; with permission.)

should be considered to eliminate all exposure to refluxate, thus liberating the patient from medical therapy.

Currently, there is no consensus on surveillance protocols following esophagus-preserving approaches. All patients require multiple surveillance endoscopies, and subsequent interventions may be required in the first year after the initial treatment. Our current follow-up protocol after RFA or EMR is to perform the first follow-up endoscopy at 6 weeks after the intervention, followed by repeat endoscopic surveillance with biopsy for the previously known length of Barrett epithelium every 3 months until the treated area is determined to be stable. In addition, subsequent ablation for areas of concern is often required during follow-up.

Recent advances in optic technology have led to the development of small-caliber endoscopes. Transnasal endoscopy using a small-caliber endoscope can be performed in the office setting without intravenous sedation, and this endoscope has a disposable sheath with an incorporated coaxial biopsy channel placed over it. Therefore, there is no need for postprocedure endoscope processing, as required for sedated endoscopy, and the cost can be significantly reduced. This technology may lead to a low-cost and safe mechanism for intensive surveillance of patients who undergo esophagus-preserving approaches.

SUMMARY

The goal of esophagus-preserving approaches for HGD and intramucosal adenocarcinoma is to provide definitive therapy while avoiding the morbidity of esophagectomy. Patient selection based on the assessment of risk factors and pretreatment clinical staging is critical (**Fig. 6**).[72] Although it is unknown whether or not long-term outcomes of the esophagus-preserving approach are comparable with those of surgical resection, esophagus-preserving approaches can be performed safely and efficiently on a select subset of patients with HGD and intramucosal adenocarcinoma. Meticulous endoscopic follow-up is required because metachronous disease can occur after endoscopic

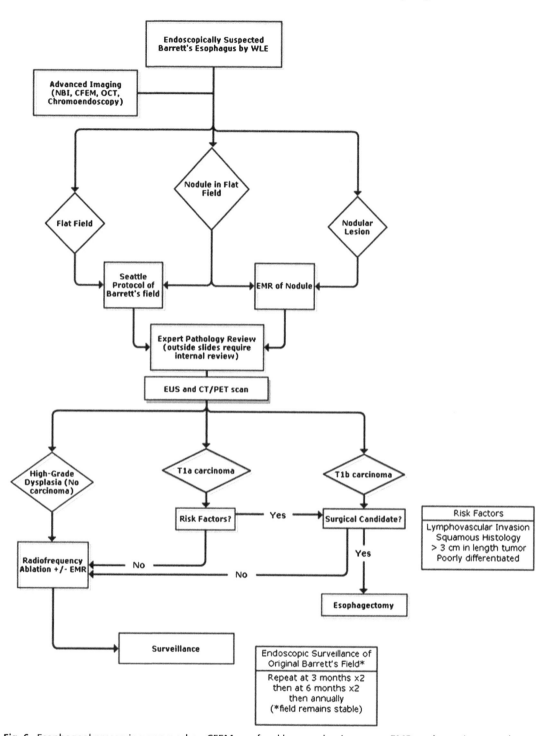

Fig. 6. Esophageal preserving approaches. CFEM, confocal laser endomicroscopy; EMR, endoscopic mucosal resection; EUS, endoscopic ultrasound; NBI, narrow band imaging; OCT, optical coherence tomography; WLE, white light endoscopy. (*From* Carr SR, Jobe BA. Esophageal preservation in the setting of high-grade dysplasia and superficial cancer. Semin Thorac Cardiovasc Surg 2010;22(2):162; with permission.)

therapies. Post-procedure, acid suppression with high-dose PPI and nocturnal H_2 blockade is a critical component for the success of esophagus-preserving approaches. Once the treated area becomes stable, a laparoscopic fundoplication should be considered to eliminate all acid exposure, thus liberating the patient from medical therapy.

REFERENCES

1. Pohl H, Sirovich B, Welch HG. Esophageal adenocarcinoma incidence: are we reaching the peak? Cancer Epidemiol Biomarkers Prev 2010;19(6):1468–70.
2. Enzinger PC, Mayer RJ. Esophageal cancer. N Engl J Med 2003;349(23):2241–52.
3. Barrett NR. The oesophagus lined by columnar epithelium. Gastroenterologia 1956;86(3):183–6.
4. Lagergren J, Bergstrom R, Lindgren A, et al. Symptomatic gastroesophageal reflux as a risk factor for esophageal adenocarcinoma. N Engl J Med 1999; 340(11):825–31.
5. Collard JM. High-grade dysplasia in Barrett's esophagus. The case for esophagectomy. Chest Surg Clin N Am 2002;12(1):77–92.
6. Falk GW, Rice TW, Goldblum JR, et al. Jumbo biopsy forceps protocol still misses unsuspected cancer in Barrett's esophagus with high-grade dysplasia. Gastrointest Endosc 1999;49(2):170–6.
7. Birkmeyer JD, Siewers AE, Finlayson EV, et al. Hospital volume and surgical mortality in the United States. N Engl J Med 2002;346(15):1128–37.
8. Orringer MB, Marshall B, Chang AC, et al. Two thousand transhiatal esophagectomies: changing trends, lessons learned. Ann Surg 2007;246(3): 363–72 [discussion: 372–4].
9. Oh DS, Hagen JA, Chandrasoma PT, et al. Clinical biology and surgical therapy of intramucosal adenocarcinoma of the esophagus. J Am Coll Surg 2006; 203(2):152–61.
10. Rice TW, Blackstone EH, Adelstein DJ, et al. Role of clinically determined depth of tumor invasion in the treatment of esophageal carcinoma. J Thorac Cardiovasc Surg 2003;125(5):1091–102.
11. Rice TW, Zuccaro G Jr, Adelstein DJ, et al. Esophageal carcinoma: depth of tumor invasion is predictive of regional lymph node status. Ann Thorac Surg 1998;65(3):787–92.
12. Fernando HC, Murthy SC, Hofstetter W, et al. The Society of Thoracic Surgeons practice guideline series: guidelines for the management of Barrett's esophagus with high-grade dysplasia. Ann Thorac Surg 2009;87(6):1993–2002.
13. Schnell TG, Sontag SJ, Chejfec G, et al. Long-term nonsurgical management of Barrett's esophagus with high-grade dysplasia. Gastroenterology 2001; 120(7):1607–19.
14. Levine DS, Haggitt RC, Blount PL, et al. An endoscopic biopsy protocol can differentiate high-grade dysplasia from early adenocarcinoma in Barrett's esophagus. Gastroenterology 1993;105(1):40–50.
15. Rice TW. Pro: esophagectomy is the treatment of choice for high-grade dysplasia in Barrett's esophagus. Am J Gastroenterol 2006;101(10):2177–9.
16. Sepesi B, Watson TJ, Zhou D, et al. Are endoscopic therapies appropriate for superficial submucosal esophageal adenocarcinoma? An analysis of esophagectomy specimens. J Am Coll Surg 2010; 210(4):418–27.
17. Buttar NS, Wang KK, Sebo TJ, et al. Extent of high-grade dysplasia in Barrett's esophagus correlates with risk of adenocarcinoma. Gastroenterology 2001;120(7):1630–9.
18. Weston AP, Sharma P, Topalovski M, et al. Long-term follow-up of Barrett's high-grade dysplasia. Am J Gastroenterol 2000;95(8):1888–93.
19. Ell C, May A, Pech O, et al. Curative endoscopic resection of early esophageal adenocarcinomas (Barrett's cancer). Gastrointest Endosc 2007;65(1): 3–10.
20. Pech O, May A, Gossner L, et al. Curative endoscopic therapy in patients with early esophageal squamous-cell carcinoma or high-grade intraepithelial neoplasia. Endoscopy 2007;39(1):30–5.
21. Stein HJ, Feith M, Bruecher BL, et al. Early esophageal cancer: pattern of lymphatic spread and prognostic factors for long-term survival after surgical resection. Ann Surg 2005;242(4):566–73 [discussion: 573–5].
22. Bolton WD, Hofstetter WL, Francis AM, et al. Impact of tumor length on long-term survival of pT1 esophageal adenocarcinoma. J Thorac Cardiovasc Surg 2009;138(4):831–6.
23. Rudolph RE, Vaughan TL, Storer BE, et al. Effect of segment length on risk for neoplastic progression in patients with Barrett esophagus. Ann Intern Med 2000;132(8):612–20.
24. Ormsby AH, Petras RE, Henricks WH, et al. Observer variation in the diagnosis of superficial oesophageal adenocarcinoma. Gut 2002;51(5):671–6.
25. Reid BJ, Haggitt RC, Rubin CE, et al. Observer variation in the diagnosis of dysplasia in Barrett's esophagus. Hum Pathol 1988;19(2):166–78.
26. Reid BJ, Blount PL, Rubin CE, et al. Flow-cytometric and histological progression to malignancy in Barrett's esophagus: prospective endoscopic surveillance of a cohort. Gastroenterology 1992;102(4 Pt 1): 1212–9.
27. Reid BJ, Levine DS, Longton G, et al. Predictors of progression to cancer in Barrett's esophagus: baseline histology and flow cytometry identify low- and high-risk patient subsets. Am J Gastroenterol 2000; 95(7):1669–76.
28. Reid BJ, Prevo LJ, Galipeau PC, et al. Predictors of progression in Barrett's esophagus II: baseline 17p (p53) loss of heterozygosity identifies a patient subset at increased risk for neoplastic progression. Am J Gastroenterol 2001;96(10):2839–48.
29. Sabo E, Beck AH, Montgomery EA, et al. Computerized morphometry as an aid in determining the grade of dysplasia and progression to adenocarcinoma in Barrett's esophagus. Lab Invest 2006; 86(12):1261–71.

30. Reddymasu SC, Sharma P. Advances in endoscopic imaging of the esophagus. Gastroenterol Clin North Am 2008;37(4):763–74, vii.

31. Stevens PD, Lightdale CJ, Green PH, et al. Combined magnification endoscopy with chromoendoscopy for the evaluation of Barrett's esophagus. Gastrointest Endosc 1994;40(6):747–9.

32. Wong Kee Song LM, Adler DG, Chand B, et al. Chromoendoscopy. Gastrointest Endosc 2007;66(4):639–49.

33. Canto MI, Setrakian S, Willis JE, et al. Methylene blue staining of dysplastic and nondysplastic Barrett's esophagus: an in vivo and ex vivo study. Endoscopy 2001;33(5):391–400.

34. Gono K, Obi T, Yamaguchi M, et al. Appearance of enhanced tissue features in narrow-band endoscopic imaging. J Biomed Opt 2004;9(3):568–77.

35. Ngamruengphong S, Sharma VK, Das A. Diagnostic yield of methylene blue chromoendoscopy for detecting specialized intestinal metaplasia and dysplasia in Barrett's esophagus: a meta-analysis. Gastrointest Endosc 2009;69(6):1021–8.

36. Guelrud M, Herrera I, Essenfeld H, et al. Enhanced magnification endoscopy: a new technique to identify specialized intestinal metaplasia in Barrett's esophagus. Gastrointest Endosc 2001;53(6):559–65.

37. Pech O, Petrone MC, Manner H, et al. One-step chromoendoscopy and structure enhancement using balsamic vinegar for screening of Barrett's esophagus. Acta Gastroenterol Belg 2008;71(2):243–5.

38. Wolfsen HC, Crook JE, Krishna M, et al. Prospective, controlled tandem endoscopy study of narrow band imaging for dysplasia detection in Barrett's esophagus. Gastroenterology 2008;135(1):24–31.

39. Curvers WL, Herrero LA, Wallace MB, et al. Endoscopic tri-modal imaging is more effective than standard endoscopy in identifying early-stage neoplasia in Barrett's esophagus. Gastroenterology 2010;139(4):1106–14.

40. Puli SR, Reddy JB, Bechtold ML, et al. Staging accuracy of esophageal cancer by endoscopic ultrasound: a meta-analysis and systematic review. World J Gastroenterol 2008;14(10):1479–90.

41. Wang TD, Van Dam J. Optical biopsy: a new frontier in endoscopic detection and diagnosis. Clin Gastroenterol Hepatol 2004;2(9):744–53.

42. Dunbar KB, Okolo P 3rd, Montgomery E, et al. Confocal laser endomicroscopy in Barrett's esophagus and endoscopically inapparent Barrett's neoplasia: a prospective, randomized, double-blind, controlled, crossover trial. Gastrointest Endosc 2009;70(4):645–54.

43. Wallace MB, Sharma P, Lightdale C, et al. Preliminary accuracy and interobserver agreement for the detection of intraepithelial neoplasia in Barrett's esophagus with probe-based confocal laser endomicroscopy. Gastrointest Endosc 2010;72(1):19–24.

44. Bajbouj M, Vieth M, Rosch T, et al. Probe-based confocal laser endomicroscopy compared with standard four-quadrant biopsy for evaluation of neoplasia in Barrett's esophagus. Endoscopy 2010;42(6):435–40.

45. Borovicka J, Fischer J, Neuweiler J, et al. Autofluorescence endoscopy in surveillance of Barrett's esophagus: a multicenter randomized trial on diagnostic efficacy. Endoscopy 2006;38(9):867–72.

46. Chemaly M, Scalone O, Durivage G, et al. Miniprobe EUS in the pretherapeutic assessment of early esophageal neoplasia. Endoscopy 2008;40(1):2–6.

47. Savoy AD, Wallace MB. EUS in the management of the patient with dysplasia in Barrett's esophagus. J Clin Gastroenterol 2005;39(4):263–7.

48. Gananadha S, Hazebroek EJ, Leibman S, et al. The utility of FDG-PET in the preoperative staging of esophageal cancer. Dis Esophagus 2008;21(5):389–94.

49. Meyers BF, Downey RJ, Decker PA, et al. The utility of positron emission tomography in staging of potentially operable carcinoma of the thoracic esophagus: results of the American College of Surgeons Oncology Group Z0060 trial. J Thorac Cardiovasc Surg 2007;133(3):738–45.

50. Gockel I, Sgourakis G, Lyros O, et al. Risk of lymph node metastasis in submucosal esophageal cancer: a review of surgically resected patients. Expert Rev Gastroenterol Hepatol 2011;5(3):371–84.

51. Overholt BF. Acid suppression and reepithelialization after ablation of Barrett's esophagus. Dig Dis 2000;18(4):232–9.

52. Litle VR, Luketich JD, Christie NA, et al. Photodynamic therapy as palliation for esophageal cancer: experience in 215 patients. Ann Thorac Surg 2003;76(5):1687–92 [discussion: 1692–3].

53. Shaheen NJ, Sharma P, Overholt BF, et al. Radiofrequency ablation in Barrett's esophagus with dysplasia. N Engl J Med 2009;360(22):2277–88.

54. Shaheen NJ, Peery AF, Hawes RH, et al. Quality of life following radiofrequency ablation of dysplastic Barrett's esophagus. Endoscopy 2010;42(10):790–9.

55. Dumot JA, Vargo JJ 2nd, Falk GW, et al. An open-label, prospective trial of cryospray ablation for Barrett's esophagus high-grade dysplasia and early esophageal cancer in high-risk patients. Gastrointest Endosc 2009;70(4):635–44.

56. Shaheen NJ, Greenwald BD, Peery AF, et al. Safety and efficacy of endoscopic spray cryotherapy for Barrett's esophagus with high-grade dysplasia. Gastrointest Endosc 2010;71(4):680–5.

57. Katada C, Muto M, Manabe T, et al. Esophageal stenosis after endoscopic mucosal resection of superficial esophageal lesions. Gastrointest Endosc 2003;57(2):165–9.

58. Seewald S, Ang TL, Omar S, et al. Endoscopic mucosal resection of early esophageal squamous

cell cancer using the Duette mucosectomy kit. Endoscopy 2006;38(10):1029–31.

59. Soehendra N, Seewald S, Groth S, et al. Use of modified multiband ligator facilitates circumferential EMR in Barrett's esophagus (with video). Gastrointest Endosc 2006;63(6):847–52.

60. May A, Gossner L, Behrens A, et al. A prospective randomized trial of two different endoscopic resection techniques for early stage cancer of the esophagus. Gastrointest Endosc 2003;58(2):167–75.

61. May A, Gossner L, Pech O, et al. Local endoscopic therapy for intraepithelial high-grade neoplasia and early adenocarcinoma in Barrett's oesophagus: acute-phase and intermediate results of a new treatment approach. Eur J Gastroenterol Hepatol 2002; 14(10):1085–91.

62. Pech O, Behrens A, May A, et al. Long-term results and risk factor analysis for recurrence after curative endoscopic therapy in 349 patients with high-grade intraepithelial neoplasia and mucosal adenocarcinoma in Barrett's oesophagus. Gut 2008;57(9):1200–6.

63. Pouw RE, Wirths K, Eisendrath P, et al. Efficacy of radiofrequency ablation combined with endoscopic resection for Barrett's esophagus with early neoplasia. Clin Gastroenterol Hepatol 2010;8(1):23–9.

64. Yamamoto H. Technology insight: endoscopic submucosal dissection of gastrointestinal neoplasms. Nat Clin Pract Gastroenterol Hepatol 2007;4(9):511–20.

65. Ono S, Fujishiro M, Niimi K, et al. Long-term outcomes of endoscopic submucosal dissection for superficial esophageal squamous cell neoplasms. Gastrointest Endosc 2009;70(5):860–6.

66. Witteman BP, Foxwell TJ, Monsheimer S, et al. Transoral endoscopic inner layer esophagectomy: management of high-grade dysplasia and superficial cancer with organ preservation. J Gastrointest Surg 2009;13(12):2104–12.

67. Akiyama H, Tsurumaru M, Ono Y, et al. Transoral esophagectomy. Surg Gynecol Obstet 1991; 173(5):399–400.

68. Badylak S, Meurling S, Chen M, et al. Resorbable bioscaffold for esophageal repair in a dog model. J Pediatr Surg 2000;35(7):1097–103.

69. Badylak SF, Vorp DA, Spievack AR, et al. Esophageal reconstruction with ECM and muscle tissue in a dog model. J Surg Res 2005;128(1):87–97.

70. Nieponice A, McGrath K, Qureshi I, et al. An extracellular matrix scaffold for esophageal stricture prevention after circumferential EMR. Gastrointest Endosc 2009;69(2):289–96.

71. Badylak SF, Hoppo T, Nieponice A, et al. Esophageal preservation in five male patients after endoscopic inner-layer circumferential resection in the setting of superficial cancer: a regenerative medicine approach with a biologic scaffold. Tissue Eng Part A 2011;17(11–12):1643–50.

72. Carr SR, Jobe BA. Esophageal preservation in the setting of high-grade dysplasia and superficial cancer. Semin Thorac Cardiovasc Surg 2010;22(2): 155–64.

Advances in the Management of Esophageal Perforation

Philip W. Carrott Jr, MD[a,1], Donald E. Low, MD, FRCS(C)[b,c,*]

KEYWORDS

- Esophageal perforation • Boerhaave syndrome • Stent
- Endoscopy

Esophageal perforation is a relatively rare surgical emergency that historically has been associated with a mortality as high as 80%.[1] For much of the twentieth century, operative therapy was considered the standard of care, with outcomes linked to management in the first 24 hours after injury. Nonsurgical management was first reported by Cameron and colleagues[2] in 1979 and has seen wider application with the evolution of endoscopic therapeutic techniques. Originally, nonsurgical management included nil by mouth, antibiotics, drainage, and postpyloric feeding, although now the use of radiologic and endoscopic techniques has expanded the management options significantly. The goals of therapy are to control the septic source, closure of the perforation, and drainage of associated contamination. Improvements in imaging technologies and critical care have likely contributed to improvements in morbidity and survival as seen in recent case series in which mortality ranges from 2% to 20% (**Table 1**).

We believe that although expeditious treatment remains an important issue, management of esophageal perforation at an experienced center with a multidisciplinary team experienced in operative management, interventional radiology, and therapeutic endoscopy is likely more important than the time frame of diagnosis and treatment of the perforation.[1] **Fig. 1** demonstrates how in our experience improved outcomes have paralleled the increased use of nonoperative therapies at our institution. This review focuses on the initial diagnosis and management and patient selection for operative and nonoperative management. We also highlight the increased application of hybrid approaches in which nonoperative and operative therapies are used concurrently or sequentially.

DIAGNOSIS

The presentation of an esophageal perforation can be diverse. The rarity of esophageal perforation is demonstrated by the fact that most reports from major referral centers contain less than 100 patients (see **Table 1**). In the United States and Europe, the most common type of perforation is iatrogenic (approximately 60% in most series), usually as part of endoscopic therapy for stricture or achalasia.[3] Barogenic or Boerhaave syndrome make up about 15% to 30% of cases, with trauma, foreign body ingestion, and operative injury accounting for most of the remaining benign

The authors have nothing to disclose.

a Department of Surgery, Virginia Mason Medical Center, 1100 Ninth Avenue, C6-GS, Seattle, WA 98111, USA
b Thoracic Oncology and Thoracic Surgery, Department of Surgery, Virginia Mason Medical Center, 1100 Ninth Avenue, C6-GS, Seattle, WA 98111, USA
c University of Washington School of Medicine, Seattle, WA, USA
1 Present address: Division of Thoracic and Cardiovascular Surgery, University of Virginia Health System, PO Box 800679, Charlottesville, VA 22908-0679.
* Corresponding author. Thoracic Oncology and Thoracic Surgery, Department of Surgery, Virginia Mason Medical Center, 1100 Ninth Avenue, C6-GS, Seattle, WA 98111.
E-mail address: gtsdel@vmmc.org

Thorac Surg Clin 21 (2011) 541–555
doi:10.1016/j.thorsurg.2011.08.002

Table 1
Recent case series documenting management of esophageal perforation

Author	Study Period	N	Management		Perforation Etiology		Mortality			LOS	
			Operative (%)	Nonoperative (%)	Iatrogenic	Spontaneous (%)	Operative (%)	Nonoperative (%)	Total (%)	Operative	Nonoperative
Muir et al[43]	1985–2000	75	58 (77)	17 (23)	56 (75)	13 (17)	8 (14)	4 (24)	12 (16)	NR	NR
Port et al[44]	1990–2001	26	21 (81)	5 (19)	19 (73)	2 (8)	1 (5)	0 (0)	1 (4)	NR	NR
Richardson[10]	1985–2004	64	64 (100)	0 (0)	34 (53)	18 (28)	1 (2)	NA	1 (2)	NR	NR
Vogel et al[17]	1992–2004	47	15 (32)	32 (68)	25 (53)	14 (30)	2 (4.7)	0 (0)	2 ()	26 d overall	
Hermansson et al[45]	1970–2006	125	99 (79)	26 (21)	70 (56)	49 (39)	20 (20)	4 (15)	24 (19)	25 d	16 d
Schmidt et al[46]	1996–2006	62	32 (52)	30 (48)	33 (53)	29 (47)	5 (16)	4 (13)	9 (15)	27 d	22 d
Eroglu et al[47]	1989–2008	44	30 (68)	14 (32)	27 (61)	2 (5)	3 (10)	2 (14)	5 (11)	23 d overall	
Vallbohmer et al[48]	1996–2008	44	24 (55)	20 (45)	28 (64)	9 (20)	2 (8)	1 (5)	3 (7)	21 d overall	
Merchea et al[28]	1996–2008	39	11 (28)	28 (72)	39 (100)	0 (0)	4 (36)	0 (0)	4 (10)	NR	NR
Keeling et al[49]	1997–2008	97	72 (74)	25 (26)	50 (51)	23 (24)	6 (8)	2 (8)	8 (8)	29 d	15 d
Abbas et al[16]	1998–2008	119	91 (76)	28 (24)	75 (63)	44 (37)	14 (15)	1 (4)	15 (13)	24 d	13 d
Kuppusamy et al[1]	1989–2009	81	48 (59)	33 (41)	51 (63)	24 (30)	1 (2)	2 (6)	3 (4)	16 d	10 d
Minnich et al[50]	1998–2009	81	52 (64)	29 (36)	35 (43)	21 (26)	6 (12)	3 (10)	9 (11)	13.5 d	9 d

Abbreviations: LOS, length of stay; NA, not applicable; NR, not reported; Total, total group, including perforations.

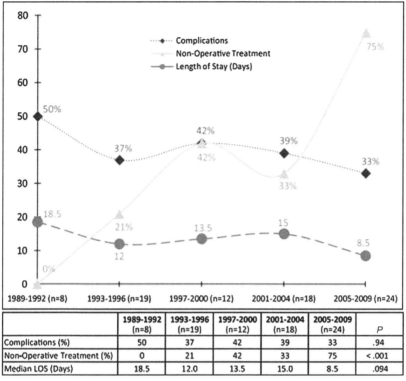

	1989-1992 (n=8)	1993-1996 (n=19)	1997-2000 (n=12)	2001-2004 (n=18)	2005-2009 (n=24)	P
Complications (%)	50	37	42	39	33	.94
Non-Operative Treatment (%)	0	21	42	33	75	< .001
Median LOS (Days)	18.5	12.0	13.5	15.0	8.5	.094

Fig. 1. Nonoperative therapy, complications, and length of stay in a series of acute esophageal perforation. (*From* Kuppusamy M, Hubka M, Felisky CD, et al. Evolving management strategies in esophageal perforation: surgeons using nonoperative techniques to improve outcomes. J Am Coll Surg 2011;213(1):164–71; with permission.)

perforations. A timely diagnosis typically offers more options in management, so a high index of suspicion on the part of the primary treating physician is needed. In our experience, 16 of 46 iatrogenic perforations (35%) were diagnosed within 2 hours, with all handled nonoperatively in the last 5 years.[1] We have developed an algorithm for the investigation and management of these patients with acute esophageal perforation, highlighting the increased use of endoscopy in both diagnosis and treatment (**Fig. 2**).

The initial assessment of the patient involves assessing physiologic stability, with the treatment and resuscitation of pain, hypotension, or sepsis being critical before proceeding to investigations of the location and extent of the perforation. The major advances in diagnosis of esophageal perforation involve greater early use of endoscopy and computed tomographic (CT) scanning to assess the location and extent of the perforation, as well as the presence of secondary pathology that often requires synchronous management and could affect the treatment of the perforation itself. In addition, assessment of the extent of mediastinal or pleural contamination is extremely important. Treatment decisions are then based on the stability

of the patient, extent of contamination on CT scan, and specific assessment of the perforation, including size, location, mucosal viability, and presence of secondary pathology.

In stable patients, we continue to recommend initiating assessment with upper gastrointestinal contrast studies, specifically water-soluble contrast, followed by barium contrast when water-soluble study results are negative. Barium contrast is more accurate than water-soluble contrast, up to 22% more in 1 prospective series of esophageal perforation.[4] Barium, however, should not be routinely used if a significant perforation is identified. Historical concerns that extraluminal barium contamination increases the degree of mediastinal or pleural inflammation are inaccurate; however, if a large volume extravasates into the chest or abdomen, artifact from the barium impairs the accuracy of subsequent CT imaging. Prospective studies quantifying the sensitivity and specificity of contrast swallow examinations are few in the literature because patient numbers tend to be small in most series. Evaluations of radiologic studies for anastomotic leak after esophagectomy show poor sensitivity and low negative predictive values (40% and 60%, respectively), with these figures improving when used in conjunction with CT and endoscopy.[5–7]

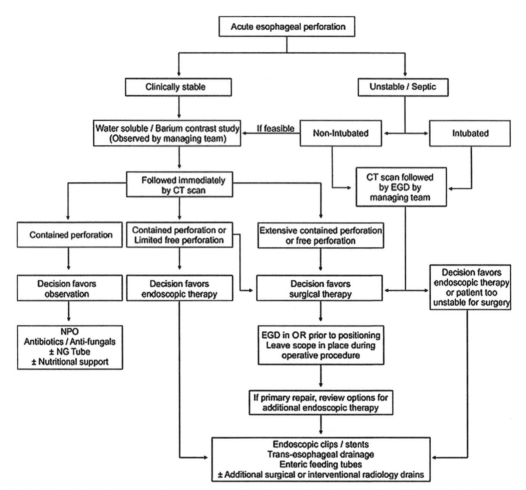

Fig. 2. Algorithm for diagnosis and management of acute esophageal perforation. CT, computed tomography; EGD, esophagogastroduodenoscopy; NG, nasogastric; NPO, nil per os; OR, operating room. (*From* Kuppusamy M, Hubka M, Felisky CD, et al. Evolving management strategies in esophageal perforation: surgeons using nonoperative techniques to improve outcomes. J Am Coll Surg 2011;213(1):164–71; with permission.)

A CT scan done immediately after the contrast studies increases the accuracy of diagnosis by demonstrating small amounts of extraluminal air, contrast, or fluid. Unless the perforation is contained and is seen to drain back into the lumen, more centers are favoring subsequent endoscopic evaluation (**Table 2**). For most iatrogenic injuries, the injury is limited, and, typically, if the injury is noted immediately, contamination of the mediastinal or pleural spaces is limited. Patients with mediastinal air only and no active leak on swallow studies are typically good candidates for endoscopic therapy or observation alone. Patients with Boerhaave syndrome, however, are more likely to be associated with extensive contamination. Sharp foreign bodies most commonly lodge in the cervical esophagus. When possible, removal of the foreign body with a flexible endoscope and overtube is recommended before assessment of the extent of

the perforation. If the foreign body can be removed endoscopically and extraluminal contamination is limited, these perforations are also often appropriate for nonsurgical management.[3] **Fig. 3** demonstrates a patient who ingested a wire with a meal, which lodged in his cervical esophagus and created a tracheoesophageal fistula. The patient presented 2 weeks later with persistent dysphagia and, on removal of the wire by a combination of bronchoscopic and endoscopic manipulation, was treated with clipping of the perforation and esophageal stenting. The patient recovered uneventfully and was discharged after a 5-day hospital stay still receiving nasojejunal tube feeds.

Endoscopy is often used as a component of evaluation of penetrating trauma to the neck, which is complicated by esophageal injury in 5% of cases. Case series in trauma patients have found a sensitivity and specificity of more than 90%, with 99%

Table 2
Use of modern technology in diagnosis and treatment of esophageal perforation

Author	Study Period	N	Diagnostic Test Use Reported in Study			Use of Therapeutic Endoscopy	MIS
			UGI	CT	EGD		
Muir et al[43]	1985–2000	75	NR	NR	NR	NR	NR
Port et al[44]	1990–2001	26	UGI	NR	NR	NR	NR
Richardson[10]	1985–2004	64	NR	NR	NR	NR	NR
Vogel et al[17]	1992–2004	47	UGI	CT	NR	NR	NR
Hermansson et al[45]	1970–2006	125	98 (78%)	22(18%)	5 (4%)	6 (5%)	NR
Schmidt et al[46]	1996–2006	62	UGI	CT	EGD	22 (35%)	NR
Eroglu et al[47]	1989–2008	44	19 (43%)	0 (0%)	25 (57%)	4 (9%)	NR
Vallbohmer et al[48]	1996–2008	44	16 (36%)	19 (43%)	26 (59%)	12 (27%)	NR
Merchea et al[28]	1996–2008	39	UGI	CT	EGD	NR	NR
Keeling et al[49]	1997–2008	97	NR	NR	32 (33%)	3 (4%)	NR
Abbas et al[16]	1998–2008	119	UGI	CT	EGD	Few	NR
Kuppusamy et al[1]	1989–2009	81	61 (75%)	46 (57%)	52 (64%)	23 (28%)	NR
Minnich et al[50]	1998–2009	81	UGI	CT	NR	5 (6%)	NR

Presence of UGI/CT/EGD in a column indicates use of that technology in diagnosis, as reported by the investigators, although incidence of use was not reported in the study.

Abbreviations: EGD, upper endoscopy; MIS, minimally invasive surgery; NR, not reported; UGI, upper gastrointestinal series.

accuracy for endoscopic assessment.[8,9] These results are much better than contrast swallow studies, which have a 10% false-negative result for assessment with barium in thoracic perforations.[9] Concerns that air insufflation associated with endoscopy worsens the contamination associated with perforation have not been conclusively demonstrated in any recent study.

TREATMENT OPTIONS FOR ACUTE ESOPHAGEAL PERFORATION

After diagnostic workup, resuscitation and monitoring for signs of sepsis continue. As stated earlier, those patients with contained perforations on upper gastrointestinal tract may undergo a trial of nil by mouth and monitoring in the hospital. The spectrum of severity of the perforation and the

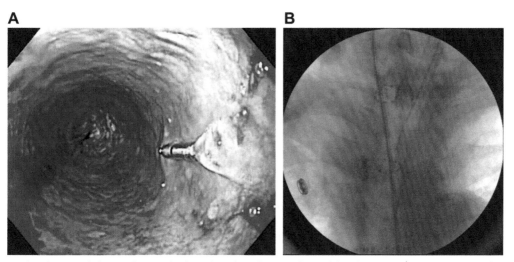

Fig. 3. Clip closure of chronic foreign body–induced tracheoesophageal fistula. Stent placement was performed after clip closure.

health status of the patient, in addition to the level of contamination with food or foreign bodies, dictate which patients are appropriate for nonoperative management. Patients with limited free perforation or an immediately identified iatrogenic perforation may do well with endoscopic therapy. Operative or hybrid treatment is typically indicated for patients with extensive perforations and large amounts of thoracic or abdominal contamination.

Series from experienced centers show an increase in the use of nonoperative management of acute esophageal perforation in recent years (see **Table 1**). Our own experience over the last 20 years supports this management, as shown in **Fig. 1**. The treatment method used will be dependent on the clinical stability of the patient and the multidisciplinary resources available to the surgical team, particularly the endoscopic expertise of the gastroenterological or surgical staff. The condition of the esophageal mucosa and the presence of secondary pathology also dictate how the perforation will be most effectively managed. We start with a discussion of operative therapy, as it remains the cornerstone of management of acute esophageal perforation since the first successful cases were reported in the late 1940s.[3]

OPERATIVE THERAPY

For many years, aggressive surgical management was mandated for esophageal perforation.[10] Current operative approaches include drainage alone; decortication and drainage; primary repair, with or without a tissue buttress; repair over a T tube to establish a controlled fistula; esophageal resection; or esophageal exclusion with cervical esophagostomy, stapling of the esophagus distally, and gastrostomy, with all these approaches usually associated with placement of a feeding jejunostomy. The operative approach selected depends on the patient's hemodynamic stability, the presence of other pathology, and the suitability of the esophageal mucosa and muscular layers for primary repair. Richardson advocates buttressing the repair or site of perforation in all cases, even if primary repair was not possible, as in a late presentation.[10,11] Many series and reviews have highlighted treatment within 24 hours as an important issue associated with a successful outcome.[3,12,13]

Operative therapy is more commonly required in free perforations with extensive mediastinal or pleural contamination. Boerhaave syndrome and larger iatrogenic perforations are most likely to benefit from operative intervention. Mortality varies widely, with a mean of 18% and range from 0% to 80% from one meta-analysis of series between 1990 and 2003.[3] More recent series may be seen

in **Table 1**, showing operative mortality of 2% to 20%, with mortality in many series below 10%.

Drainage alone is typically used when the patient is unstable and more elaborate operations are not feasible or in patients presenting late, often after previous treatment, and when the perforation is inadequately drained. Decortication is often required in patients with extensive collapsed lung and intrapleural contamination. Primary repair should be performed in most cases in which there are a sizable perforation and healthy esophageal tissues. The size and location of the perforation dictate whether the approach is cervical, thoracic, or abdominal. In general, perforations are reapproximated and closed simply in 1 or 2 layers. Primary repair can also be facilitated by endoscopic guidance.[14] Buttressing of primary repairs can be achieved using pleura, pericardial fat, intercostal or diaphragmatic muscle flap, stomach, or omentum.

Establishing a controlled fistula with a T tube is desirable if the diagnosis has been delayed and repair is not feasible because of extensive damage to the esophageal mucosa and muscular wall, which necessitates esophageal narrowing with primary closure. T tubes may also be used in patients who are profoundly unstable at the time of surgery.

Esophagectomy should usually be reserved for stable patients who sustain perforation to nondisseminated cancers. Esophageal exclusion should be reserved for the nonviable esophagus that cannot be repaired or if the patient's hemodynamic stability or secondary pathology precludes primary repair. Exclusion is sometimes overused in centers with less experience in the management of acute esophageal perforation. Esophageal exclusion is typically not appropriate in the severely unstable patient. In this situation, appropriate drainage with jejunal and gastric enteric access for feeding and/or drainage usually provides adequate initial therapy, allowing the patient to be stabilized.

Several reports have focused on the advantages of aggressive operative management in Boerhaave syndrome.[11] Sutcliffe and colleagues[15] treated 21 patients with Boerhaave syndrome from 2001 to 2007, 10 presenting within 24 hours and 11 presenting after 24 hours. All in the early group and 7 of 11 in the late group underwent surgery on arrival. Of the 4 patients initially treated nonoperatively, 3 died, and 2 of these patients underwent esophageal exclusion before dying. The investigators' conclusions that Boerhaave syndrome should be treated with an exclusively surgical approach, no matter what the time from injury, should be assessed in light of the success achieved with selective surgical or endoscopic therapy reported in several other case series (see **Tables 1** and **2**).

Neel and colleagues[11] reviewed 31 patients presenting with Boerhaave syndrome, 25 of whom had uncontained extravasation on initial contrast study. Of these patients, 24 were taken for operative repair, regardless of time since perforation. The investigators report successful closure with a combination of primary repair and buttressing with tissue flaps in all cases. Although outcomes were good for the entire series, the earlier treatment group showed less complications (25% vs 50%) and shorter length of stay (8 vs 12 days). In patients initially treated nonoperatively, 4 of 6 needed subsequent operative therapy in the form of decortication.

Abbas and colleagues[16] have published the largest modern single-institution experience with acute esophageal perforation. The investigators reviewed their experience of 119 esophageal perforations over an 11-year period, including 44 patients with Boerhaave syndrome. Most patients with Boerhaave syndrome were treated operatively (34/44, 77%), all with primary repair. Outcomes in the investigators' entire series favored nonoperative management, although the patients managed nonoperatively had fewer documented comorbidities and signs of sepsis.[16] Median lengths of stay and complications were 24 days and 62% and 13 days and 36% in the operative and nonoperative groups, respectively. These investigators also analyzed their operative approaches with regard to outcomes and found that repair of perforations over a drain (eg, T tube repair) had a higher mortality than primary repair (18% vs 3%). Patients with Boerhaave syndrome did even worse with T tube repair, with a mortality of 39%. With these outcomes, the investigators advocated primary repair in patients with signs of sepsis and an uncontained leak.

In contrast, Vogel and colleagues[17] reported on a predominantly nonoperative series with 32 of 47 patients having aggressive conservative treatment. Only 1 of 14 patients with Boerhaave syndrome received an operation for the perforation, although 3 underwent delayed surgical drainage. The remainder underwent radiologically guided drain placement when indicated. Although the investigators do not report on the time to diagnosis, average length of stay in the Boerhaave syndrome group was 41 days, which is longer than reported by other, predominantly operative, series for Boerhaave syndrome in which length of stay ranged between 12 and 24 days (see **Table 1**).[11,16] The investigators' initial treatment included aggressive drainage, although they also do not describe the use of endoscopic therapies, which is an integral component of the algorithm from the same center in a subsequent report.[1,18] These series highlight the fact that one treatment approach, operative or nonoperative, does not fit every patient.

MINIMALLY INVASIVE SURGERY

Minimally invasive surgery is being increasingly applied in selected patients with acute esophageal perforation. This technique is most often reserved for stable patients with mild contamination. Reports in the literature are confined to case reports and small case series, which outline thoracoscopic and laparoscopic approaches, with most describing treatment of Boerhaave syndrome and repair of perforation caused by balloon dilation in achalasia.[19–26] Cho and colleagues[21] report a series of 15 patients with Boerhaave syndrome treated with thoracoscopy or thoracotomy, depending on the surgeon's preference. The 7 patients in the thoracoscopic group were more hemodynamically stable and demonstrated shorter operative times, less prolonged ventilation, and less mortality. Fiscon and colleagues[27] highlight the utility of both minimally invasive operative therapy and endoscopic therapy in a case report. Their patient was admitted with retrosternal chest pain after emesis, and a CT scan showed a left pleural effusion and pneumomediastinum. An endoscopy in the operating room revealed a perforation, and the patient then underwent closure and pleural flap reinforcement by left thoracoscopy. On postoperative day 6, a leak was suspected and confirmed endoscopically and subsequently closed with endoclips.

Minimally invasive treatment of perforations occurring in patients undergoing balloon dilation for achalasia is an obvious extension of current practice. When a mucosal perforation is made during a laparoscopic Heller myotomy, the perforation is closed and buttressed. Bell[20] first described this practice for patients with perforation after pneumatic dilation. A more recent publication by Sanchez-Pernaute and colleagues[25] describes their experience with 5 patients over 5 years, all treated in the same manner with closure, contralateral myotomy, and buttressing with stomach. The investigators had only 1 radiographic leak at postoperative day 6, which did not require intervention. The laparoscopic approach may offer better visualization because the location of the perforation is typically at the posterior lateral aspect of the esophagus, posterior to the angle of His.[25]

ENDOSCOPIC THERAPY

Endoscopic therapy is being increasingly used in patients whose perforation is diagnosed immediately without any signs of sepsis. Endoscopic treatment may also be appropriate in patients who are transferred stable with ongoing incompletely treated perforations. There are multiple case series of esophageal stenting in perforation and esophageal anastomotic leak. **Table 3** shows the data on stenting in patients with perforation (the anastomotic leak data were removed for clarity). Reported results are generally good, although there is a relatively wide range of mortality and length of stay. From our own data, endoscopy improved diagnosis and treatment in patients with acute esophageal perforation.[14] We separately analyzed patients in our larger series that had endoscopy as a component of diagnosis or treatment. In 10 of 21 (48%) patients who underwent endoscopy in the operating room, we found secondary pathology, for example, untreated stricture or undiagnosed malignancy, and, in 25% of these patients, endoscopic findings changed the initial planned management.[14] The ability to combine both diagnosis and treatment has certainly elevated the role of endoscopy in many upper gastrointestinal conditions. Endoscopic assessment and treatment are seeing increased application as documented in our experience, where endoscopy was used in 37% in 1990 to 1994 but increased to 80% in 2005 to 2009.[1]

Endoscopic options for treating a variety of clinical conditions continue to expand. As these endoscopic techniques are increasingly applied to treat conditions such as Barrett esophagus, achalasia, and gastroesophageal reflux disease, the potential for iatrogenic perforations increases. Pneumatic dilation for achalasia has the highest incidence of perforation at 3% to 6%, sclerotherapy for varices has a rate of perforation of 1% to 3%, and dilation for stricture after endoscopic mucosal resection for squamous cell cancer also has a rate of perforation of 1.1%.[3,9] For purely diagnostic endoscopy, perforation is rare, with an incidence of 0.03%.[28] Several case reports of iatrogenic injuries describe immediate stenting or clipping of the injury.[29,30] In these cases, drainage was not necessary because the perforation was associated with minimal to no contamination. There is no evidence to suggest that diagnostic or therapeutic endoscopy in patients with acute esophageal perforation increases the associated mediastinal or pleural contamination.

Table 3
Stenting in perforation, current case series

Study	Author Discipline	Perforations (n)	Perf Type I/S	Success (%)	Migration Rate (%)	Mortality (%)	LOS (d)	Types of Stents
Segalin et al,[37] 1996	Surgery	2	0/2	100	NR	0	NR	Wilson-Cook
Ott et al,[51] 2007	GI	4	3/1	50	33	50	NR	PolyFlex
Freeman et al,[52] 2007	Surgery	17	17/0	94	18	0	5	PolyFlex
Tuebergen et al,[53] 2008	Surgery	8	4/4	87	6	NR	NR	Ultraflex/ PolyFlex
Kim et al,[54] 2008	Surgery	9	5/4	77	35	11	19	Salivary bypass
Leers et al,[55] 2009	Surgery	9	9/0	100	3	0	6	Ultraflex
Dai et al,[31] 2011	Surgery	6	5/1	83	35	17	35	PolyFlex
van Heel et al,[33] 2010	GI	31	19/10	74	33	15	NR	Ultraflex/ PolyFlex
Ben-David et al,[18] 2011	Surgery	11 (8)[a]	NR	100	38	NR	15	NR
Kuppusamy et al,[14] 2011	Surgery/GI	52 (14)[a]	7/7	100	21[b]	0	20	PolyFlex/ Niti-S/ WallFlex

Abbreviations: GI, gastroenterology; I, iatrogenic; LOS, length of stay; NR, not reported; Perf, perforation; S, spontaneous, predominantly Boerhaave syndrome.
[a] Denotes number of patients treated with a stent out of a larger series.
[b] Unpublished data.

ENDOLUMINAL STENTING

Esophageal stenting began with malignant strictures in the early 1990s. Since that time, partially covered and now fully covered stents have been used for benign indications. Small series of stents placed for perforation and anastomotic leaks or fistulas show the potential for nonsurgical treatment in selected patients (see **Table 3**). Many of these series come from surgical groups, indicating a shift toward more interventional endoscopic experience among surgeons. The success rates in primary sealing of the perforation are good overall, although it is especially difficult to stratify patients by timing and severity of presentation. The overall experience of the managing team is key in using nonoperative approaches and endoscopic measures appropriately. Ideally, surgeons should be consulted when nonsurgical management of acute esophageal perforation is contemplated. The management of these patients is often unpredictable, and we have found that the most effective management strategy involves an interdisciplinary discussion of treatment options individualized to the condition of the patient and the individual characteristics of the perforation.

There is a variety of covered stainless steel or nitinol stents that are Food and Drug Administration (FDA) approved for malignant strictures. The PolyFlex stent (Boston Scientific, Natick, MA, USA) is a silicone-covered polyester and the only stent that is FDA approved for late removal. Two recent reports, including the largest experience using stents in acute perforations, outlined successful use of the PolyFlex in 83% of patients with benign and malignant perforations.[31,32] van Heel and colleagues[33] reported the largest series of stenting benign perforations, including 10 patients with Boerhaave syndrome, in which healing of the perforation occurred in 23 of 33 patients, but there was an overall perforation-related mortality of 21%, most often secondary to ongoing sepsis. This experience confirms that nonoperative therapy is not appropriate in all patients.

Using stents in patients with Boerhaave syndrome is more controversial not only because of increased mediastinal or pleural contamination but also because the esophagus is more likely to be normal before injury; therefore, stents have a higher incidence of migration in these patients than in those with a preexisting stricture.

Migration of endoscopically placed esophageal stents is a common problem because even stents showing no leak on confirmatory swallow study may dislodge over time. The migration rate in recent series is between 3% and 38% (see **Table 3**), with many series reporting migration of around 30%.[34] Using the appropriate stent size and refraining when possible from crossing the lower esophageal sphincter minimize migration.[35] Endoscopically clipping (**Fig. 4**) the serrated edges of the stent or transcervical or transnasal suture fixation has been used with some success in decreasing migration rates.[36] The PolyFlex and ALIMAXX (Merit Medical Systems, Inc, South Jordan, UT, USA) stents also use the woven polyester or metal struts on the exterior of the stent to provide surface friction to minimize movement.

Stenting in benign disease was initially performed for chronic fistulas as a late therapy.[37] We have also treated several patients presenting after stabilization, at an outside institution, who were referred with a persistent leak from their perforation. An example is the patient in **Fig. 4**

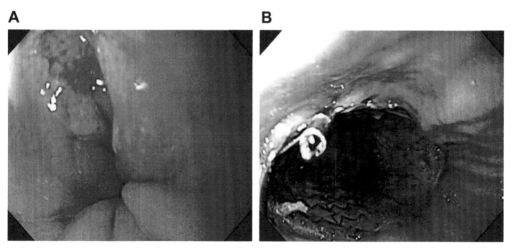

Fig. 4. Endoscopic views of perforation and surrounding lower esophageal sphincter (*A*), and successfully placed ALIMAXX stent (Merit Medical Systems, Inc, South Jordan, UT, USA) secured with an endoscopic clip (*B*).

who had a recognized perforation from pneumatic dilation for achalasia, with left-sided pleural communication. The patient underwent attempted repair at the outside hospital, which was unsuccessful. He was transferred 10 days after the perforation. Endoscopy showed healthy tissues around the leak, so a covered metal stent was deployed and clipped in place, which resolved the leak. In addition, an operative drain was upsized under fluoroscopic guidance, which effectively drained the residual contaminated left pleural cavity and allowed the patient to be discharged 7 days later.

Other fully covered metal stents are currently not FDA approved for late removal but have seen some off-label application for benign perforations (see **Table 3**). Fully covered biodegradable stents are approved in Europe and Japan made of polydioxanone or poly-l-lactic acid.[35,38] Case reports have been encouraging, and, although these stents are not yet approved for use in the United States, not requiring additional endoscopies to evaluate or remove the stent after treatment of selected perforations has obvious advantages in terms of cost and time savings.

Stent placement is typically performed with endoscopic and fluoroscopic guidance, so that the lesion in question may be visualized while deployment is monitored under fluoroscopy. The placement of esophageal stents is outside the scope of this review, but examples of stents that are currently FDA approved for esophageal use may be found in **Fig. 5**. The PolyFlex and WallFlex (Boston Scientific, Natick, MA, USA) are commonly used for benign indications, although the Evolution (Cook Medical, Bloomington, IN, USA), ALIMAXX, and Niti-S (Taewoong Medical, Gyeonggi-Do, South Korea) are also indicated for managing benign disease, and many series are reporting use and removal of these stents in perforation, although late removal of these stents is still considered off-label use.

ENDOSCOPIC CLIPS

Endoscopic clips are currently the only endoluminal device available for closure of a mucosal defect associated with acute esophageal perforation. There are 2 types of clip available that are approved by the FDA for closure of perforations that are less than 2 cm in size. The second-generation Resolution clip (Boston Scientific, Natick, MA, USA) is a through-the-scope single-use deployment clip that has been used for several years for hemostasis and mucosal tears (**Fig. 6**). Qadeer and colleagues[39] pooled case reports of endoscopic clip therapy for esophageal

perforation and found 17 patients treated by 12 centers from around the world. Perforations were treated immediately to days, weeks, or years after perforation. Chronic fistulas treated with clips were debrided before closure, with all closing between 14 and 63 days. Small iatrogenic perforations recognized immediately are candidates for consideration of endoscopic clip placement. In selected cases, clips and stents can be used together. Swallow studies should be performed to ensure control of the perforation, and any significant undrained mediastinal or pleural fluid must be separately drained.

A newer larger clip system, the OTSC (Over-The-Scope-Clip, Ovesco Endoscopy USA, Campbell, CA, USA), was approved by the FDA in December 2010. This clip attaches over the end of the endoscope and forms a crescent clip, 11 to 14 mm wide, with atraumatic or penetrating teeth (**Fig. 7**). Tissue is aspirated into the cap at the end of the endoscope or pulled in with tissue forceps, and the clip is deployed from the attached over-the-scope system. Kirschniak and colleagues[40] report a case series of more than 50 patients using the clips in the upper and lower gastrointestinal tract. Closure of 11 perforations, 7 of which were classified as upper gastrointestinal tract, was successful and without recurrence. The primary advantage of using this clip is the width of the system, allowing 1 clip to close the mucosa rather than 4 or 5 smaller clips.

DRAINAGE AND VACUUM THERAPY

Appropriate drainage of extraluminal contamination is essential to the success of any treatment approach for acute esophageal perforation. This drainage may be accomplished with either open or minimally invasive surgery or interventional radiology. In addition, there have been preliminary reports detailing endoluminal drainage through both a nasal sump tube or with the use of a vacuum-assisted closure (V.A.C., Kinetic Concepts, Inc, San Antonio, TX, USA) sponge system, as is currently used to close soft tissue defects. The reports of endoluminal vacuum-assisted closure therapy have typically involved stable patients who had persistent perianastomotic defects or fistulas after esophageal resection. Weidenhagen and colleagues[41] report a case series of patients with a median anastomotic dehiscence of 41.5%, median Acute Physiology and Chronic Health Evaluation II score of 24.5, and median time before vacuum-assisted closure therapy of 24.5 days. Of 6 patients, the leak healed in 5 using this approach, who were then discharged. Wedemeyer and colleagues[42] also documented a small

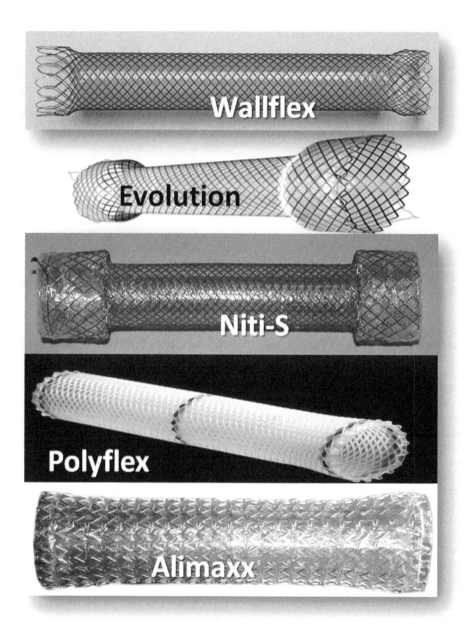

Fig. 5. FDA-approved stents for benign diseases.

series of patients principally with leaks after total gastrectomy and esophagojejunostomy who were treated with a similar system. This approach has been used principally in chronic fistulas, although application in a more acute esophageal perforation, especially associated with delayed management of ongoing leaks, may be appropriate.

HYBRID PROCEDURES

Use of endoscopic or radiologic techniques and minimally invasive or open surgery together is the most specific expression of how treatment techniques in acute esophageal perforation have evolved to improve outcomes, including morbidity and mortality. This evolution can involve interventional radiologic techniques to place chest and mediastinal drains in patients who have loculated abscesses or undrained fluid collections after primary repair. Alternatively, thoracoscopic or laparoscopic approaches can be used to place drains or decorticate lung in conjunction with endoscopic methods, that is, stents or clips, to close the perforation. **Tables 2** and **3** show that both diagnosis

A   **B**

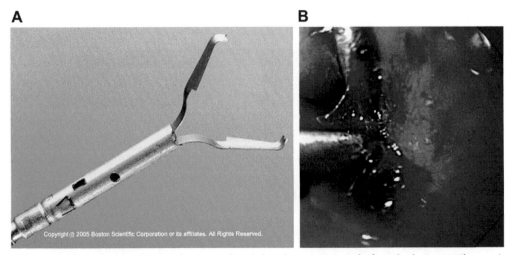

Copyright © 2005 Boston Scientific Corporation or its affiliates. All Rights Reserved.

Fig. 6. (*A*) Resolution clip. The clip may be opened and closed up to 5 times before deployment. The maximum jaw width is 11 mm. (*B*) The clips are shown closing a cervical esophageal perforation. (*Courtesy of* Boston Scientific; with permission [*A*].)

and treatment are evolving and will likely continue to do so. In 8 of the 13 series, including our own, endoscopy was used for acute assessment. This evolution has also translated into an increased application in the use of therapeutic endoscopic approaches, with the vast majority of these interventions being esophageal stents.

Ben-David and colleagues[18] treated patients prospectively according to a treatment algorithm that used both endoscopic and operative treatment according to the timing and size of the perforation. In their series of 11 patients, most perforations were small and iatrogenic, thus 8 of 11 patients were treated primarily with endoscopic stenting, and only 1 patient underwent operative repair laparoscopically. No patient was reported to need further treatment, and stents were removed 2 weeks after hospital discharge. This hybrid approach emphasizes primary endoscopic therapy, typically in small perforations that have

minimal thoracic spillage. All patients with uncontained leaks in this series also had laparoscopically placed gastrostomy and jejunostomy tubes.

We have found that intraoperative endoscopy can greatly facilitate operative repair. Specifically, this technique can guide the surgeon to the specific site of perforation, which can be challenging because of extensive mediastinal contamination and hematoma. Endoscopy can also provide the opportunity to use endoscopic techniques at the time of surgery, guide the placement of surgical sutures, and test the repair with insufflation when complete. We advocate endoscopy in the operating room after anesthesia induction but before positioning. This mode of use can allow for a more accurate operative plan and may influence whether a thoracic or abdominal approach is used. Once complete, the endoscope is left in place and serves as a guide for dissection of the esophagus and localizing the full extent of the

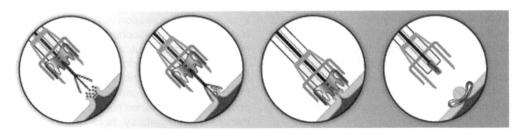

Fig. 7. The OTSC (Over-The-Scope-Clip) by Ovesco Endoscopy AG (Campbell, CA, USA). The clip is deployed by the user once the tissue in question has been aspirated into the scope or held in position by a through-the-scope grasper. (*Courtesy of* Ovesco Endoscopy AG; with permission; and *From* Ovesco.com. Available at: http://www. ovesco.com/products/20101027_OV_OTSC_eng_vND_Korr.pdf.)

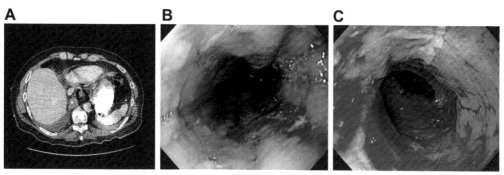

Fig. 8. (*A*) CT scan showing free mediastinal air and barium contrast in the stomach. This patient underwent endoscopy showing injury and a stricture distal to the perforation. The perforation is shown before (*B*) and after (*C*) dilation with a balloon.

perforation. Other adjuncts such as endoscopically placed feeding tubes may also be used as appropriate.

In our experience, hybrid procedures are being used more commonly.[1] This procedure can take the form of endoscopic stenting done in conjunction with primary repair or open or thoracoscopic decortication. One patient had nasomediastinal drain placement concurrent with open surgical drainage. In another example, shown in **Fig. 8**, a patient with an early diagnosis of Boerhaave syndrome was taken to the operating room and first had an endoscopy performed, showing the perforation and a proximal stricture. The stricture was dilated endoscopically, and, after open transabdominal repair of the perforation was completed, a stent was placed across the perforation and the stricture. Perforations at the gastroesophageal junction are more difficult to stent and, if approached laparoscopically, may be closed directly and reinforced with a Dor or Toupet fundoplication. Intraoperative endoscopy is important in this instance to ensure that the extent of the perforation is fully appreciated and that the esophageal repair is complete.

SUMMARY

Appropriate therapy in esophageal perforation is evolving as technology in imaging and endoscopic techniques continue to improve. More accurate diagnosis and less-invasive treatment are reducing morbidity and mortality to more acceptable levels. Endoscopic therapies should typically be used in stable patients for smaller perforations that are either contained or well drained by open or closed drains. Even long-term esophageal fistulas from perforation have closed with endoscopic therapy. Operative therapy is required in patients with large uncontained perforations and extensive contamination. Hybrid procedures that combine treatment modalities will become more common as endoscopic and radiologic therapeutic techniques continue to evolve.

REFERENCES

1. Kuppusamy M, Hubka M, Felisky CD, et al. Evolving management strategies in esophageal perforation: surgeons using nonoperative techniques to improve outcomes. J Am Coll Surg 2011;213(1):164–71.
2. Cameron JL, Kieffer RF, Hendrix TR, et al. Selective nonoperative management of contained intrathoracic esophageal disruptions. Ann Thorac Surg 1979;27:404–8.
3. Brinster CJ, Singhal S, Lee L, et al. Evolving options in the management of esophageal perforation. Ann Thorac Surg 2004;77:1475–83.
4. Buecker A, Wein BB, Neuerburg JM, et al. Esophageal perforation: comparison of use of aqueous and barium-containing contrast media. Radiology 1997;202:683–6.
5. Hogan BA, Winter DC, Broe D, et al. Prospective trial comparing contrast swallow, computed tomography and endoscopy to identify anastomotic leak following oesophagogastric surgery. Surg Endosc 2008;22:767–71.
6. Strauss C, Mal F, Perniceni T, et al. Computed tomography versus water-soluble contrast swallow in the detection of intrathoracic anastomotic leak complicating esophagogastrectomy (Ivor Lewis): a prospective study in 97 patients. Ann Surg 2010;251:647–51.
7. Tirnaksiz MB, Deschamps C, Allen MS, et al. Effectiveness of screening aqueous contrast swallow in detecting clinically significant anastomotic leaks after esophagectomy. Eur Surg Res 2005;37:123–8.
8. Arantes V, Campolina C, Valerio SH, et al. Flexible esophagoscopy as a diagnostic tool for traumatic esophageal injuries. J Trauma 2009;66:1677–82.
9. Wu JT, Mattox KL, Wall MJ Jr. Esophageal perforations: new perspectives and treatment paradigms. J Trauma 2007;63:1173–84.

10. Richardson JD. Management of esophageal perforations: the value of aggressive surgical treatment. Am J Surg 2005;190:161–5.

11. Neel D, Davis EG, Farmer R, et al. Aggressive operative treatment for emetogenic rupture yields superior results. Am Surg 2010;76:865–8.

12. Attar S, Hankins JR, Suter CM, et al. Esophageal perforation: a therapeutic challenge. Ann Thorac Surg 1990;50:45–9.

13. Lawrence DR, Moxon RE, Fountain SW, et al. Iatrogenic oesophageal perforations: a clinical review. Ann R Coll Surg Engl 1998;80:115–8.

14. Kuppusamy M, Felisky CD, Kozarek R, et al. Impact of endoscopic assessment and treatment on operative and non-operative management of acute oesophageal perforation. Br J Surg 2011;98(6):818–24.

15. Sutcliffe RP, Forshaw MJ, Datta G, et al. Surgical management of Boerhaave's syndrome in a tertiary oesophagogastric centre. Ann R Coll Surg Engl 2009;91:374–80.

16. Abbas G, Schuchert MJ, Pettiford BL, et al. Contemporaneous management of esophageal perforation. Surgery 2009;146:749–55.

17. Vogel SB, Rout WR, Martin TD, et al. Esophageal perforation in adults: aggressive, conservative treatment lowers morbidity and mortality. Ann Surg 2005;241:1016–21.

18. Ben-David K, Lopes J, Hochwald S, et al. Minimally invasive treatment of esophageal perforation using a multidisciplinary treatment algorithm: a case series. Endoscopy 2011;43:160–2.

19. Ashrafi AS, Awais O, Alvelo-Rivera M. Minimally invasive management of Boerhaave's syndrome. Ann Thorac Surg 2007;83:317–9.

20. Bell RC. Laparoscopic closure of esophageal perforation following pneumatic dilatation for achalasia. Report of two cases. Surg Endosc 1997;11:476–8.

21. Cho JS, Kim YD, Kim JW, et al. Thoracoscopic primary esophageal repair in patients with Boerhaave's syndrome. Ann Thorac Surg 2011;91:1552–5.

22. Collins C, Arumugasamy M, Larkin J, et al. Thoracoscopic repair of instrumental perforation of the oesophagus: first report. Ir J Med Sci 2002;171:68–70.

23. Hunt DR, Wills VL, Weis B, et al. Management of esophageal perforation after pneumatic dilation for achalasia. J Gastrointest Surg 2000;4:411–5.

24. Landen S, El Nakadi I. Minimally invasive approach to Boerhaave's syndrome: a pilot study of three cases. Surg Endosc 2002;16:1354–7.

25. Sanchez-Pernaute A, Aguirre EP, Talavera P, et al. Laparoscopic approach to esophageal perforation secondary to pneumatic dilation for achalasia. Surg Endosc 2009;23:1106–9.

26. Toelen C, Hendrickx L, Van HR. Laparoscopic treatment of Boerhaave's syndrome: a case report and review of the literature. Acta Chir Belg 2007;107:402–4.

27. Fiscon V, Portale G, Fania P, et al. Successful minimally invasive repair of spontaneous esophageal perforation. J Laparoendosc Adv Surg Tech A 2008;18:721–2.

28. Merchea A, Cullinane DC, Sawyer MD, et al. Esophagogastroduodenoscopy-associated gastrointestinal perforations: a single-center experience. Surgery 2010;148:876–80.

29. Hu HT, Song HY, Kim JH. Immediate placement of a temporary covered stent for the management of iatrogenic malignant esophageal perforation. Cardiovasc Intervent Radiol 2011;34(4):886–8.

30. Martinek J, Kovacova S, Nosek V, et al. Successful endoscopic treatment (clipping) of esophageal perforation during balloon dilatation in a patient with achalasia. Endoscopy 2008;40(Suppl 2):E61–62.

31. Dai Y, Chopra S, Kneif S, et al. Management of esophageal anastomotic leaks, perforations, and fistulae with self-expanding plastic stents. J Thorac Cardiovasc Surg 2011;141(5):1213–7.

32. Karbowski M, Schembre D, Kozarek R, et al. Polyflex self-expanding, removable plastic stents: assessment of treatment efficacy and safety in a variety of benign and malignant conditions of the esophagus. Surg Endosc 2008;22:1326–33.

33. van Heel NC, Haringsma J, Spaander MC, et al. Short-term esophageal stenting in the management of benign perforations. Am J Gastroenterol 2010;105:1515–20.

34. Wong RF, Adler DG, Hilden K, et al. Retrievable esophageal stents for benign indications. Dig Dis Sci 2008;53:322–9.

35. Sharma P, Kozarek R. Role of esophageal stents in benign and malignant diseases. Am J Gastroenterol 2010;105:258–73.

36. Blackmon SH, Santora R, Schwarz P, et al. Utility of removable esophageal covered self-expanding metal stents for leak and fistula management. Ann Thorac Surg 2010;89:931–6.

37. Segalin A, Bonavina L, Lazzerini M, et al. Endoscopic management of inveterate esophageal perforations and leaks. Surg Endosc 1996;10:928–32.

38. Cerna M, Kocher M, Valek V, et al. Covered biodegradable stent: new therapeutic option for the management of esophageal perforation or anastomotic leak. Cardiovasc Intervent Radiol 2011. [Epub ahead of print].

39. Qadeer MA, Dumot JA, Vargo JJ, et al. Endoscopic clips for closing esophageal perforations: case report and pooled analysis. Gastrointest Endosc 2007;66:605–11.

40. Kirschniak A, Subotova N, Zieker D, et al. The Over-The-Scope Clip (OTSC) for the treatment of gastrointestinal bleeding, perforations, and fistulas. Surg Endosc 2011;25(9):2901–5.

41. Weidenhagen R, Hartl WH, Gruetzner KU, et al. Anastomotic leakage after esophageal resection:

new treatment options by endoluminal vacuum therapy. Ann Thorac Surg 2010;90:1674–81.

42. Wedemeyer J, Brangewitz M, Kubicka S, et al. Management of major postsurgical gastroesophageal intrathoracic leaks with an endoscopic vacuum-assisted closure system. Gastrointest Endosc 2010;71:382–6.

43. Muir AD, White J, McGuigan JA, et al. Treatment and outcomes of oesophageal perforation in a tertiary referral centre. Eur J Cardiothorac Surg 2003;23: 799–804.

44. Port JL, Kent MS, Korst RJ, et al. Thoracic esophageal perforations: a decade of experience. Ann Thorac Surg 2003;75:1071–4.

45. Hermansson M, Johansson J, Gudbjartsson T, et al. Esophageal perforation in South of Sweden: results of surgical treatment in 125 consecutive patients. BMC Surg 2010;10:31.

46. Schmidt SC, Strauch S, Rosch T, et al. Management of esophageal perforations. Surg Endosc 2010;24: 2809–13.

47. Eroglu A, Turkyilmaz A, Aydin Y, et al. Current management of esophageal perforation: 20 years experience. Dis Esophagus 2009;22:374–80.

48. Vallbohmer D, Holscher AH, Holscher M, et al. Options in the management of esophageal perforation: analysis over a 12-year period. Dis Esophagus 2010;23:185–90.

49. Keeling WB, Miller DL, Lam GT, et al. Low mortality after treatment for esophageal perforation: a single-center experience. Ann Thorac Surg 2010;90:1669–73.

50. Minnich DJ, Yu P, Bryant AS, et al. Management of thoracic esophageal perforations. Eur J Cardiothorac Surg 2011. [Epub ahead of print].

51. Ott C, Ratiu N, Endlicher E, et al. Self-expanding Polyflex plastic stents in esophageal disease: various indications, complications, and outcomes. Surg Endosc 2007;21:889–96.

52. Freeman RK, Ascioti AJ, Wozniak TC. Postoperative esophageal leak management with the Polyflex esophageal stent. J Thorac Cardiovasc Surg 2007; 133:333–8.

53. Tuebergen D, Rijcken E, Mennigen R, et al. Treatment of thoracic esophageal anastomotic leaks and esophageal perforations with endoluminal stents: efficacy and current limitations. J Gastrointest Surg 2008;12:1168–76.

54. Kim AW, Liptay MJ, Snow N, et al. Utility of silicone esophageal bypass stents in the management of delayed complex esophageal disruptions. Ann Thorac Surg 2008;85:1962–7.

55. Leers JM, Vivaldi C, Schafer H, et al. Endoscopic therapy for esophageal perforation or anastomotic leak with a self-expandable metallic stent. Surg Endosc 2009;23:2258–62.

New Pharmacologic Approaches in Gastroesophageal Reflux Disease

David Armstrong, MA, MB BChir, FRCP(UK), AGAF, FRCPC[a],
Daniel Sifrim, MD, PhD[b],*

KEYWORDS

- Gastroesophageal reflux disease • GERD
- Pharmacologic therapies • Heartburn

Gastroesophageal reflux disease (GERD) has come to be regarded as a simple condition that is easy to treat; proton pump inhibitors (PPIs) are generally considered the most effective medical treatment of GERD. Patients with mild or infrequent symptoms often do not require PPI therapy but those with more severe or frequent symptoms may benefit significantly from regular PPI therapy.

One of the major challenges in GERD management is the persistence of symptoms despite regular, once-daily therapy, considered by some as PPI failure. However, this is not necessarily a failure of acid suppression therapy. Current, first-generation PPIs have a short plasma half-life and cannot provide day-long acid suppression; thus, there are opportunities for improved outcomes with (1) more frequent dosing using current PPIs, (2) longer-acting PPIs or potassium-competitive acid blockers (P-CABs), (3) antireflux agents, (4) visceral pain modulators, or (5) mucosal protectants. In the short-term, improved outcomes can be achieved by fine-tuning treatment using currently available medications, based on their pharmacology and the patient's disease manifestations; a careful consideration of the choice of drug, dose, and treatment regimen is crucial in the day-to-day management of GERD. For the future, an improved understanding of GERD and the pharmacology of available medications is essential for improving symptoms and quality of life.

BACKGROUND

The prevalence of GERD is increasing worldwide and it has become the most prevalent gastrointestinal disorder. It is responsible for a substantial proportion of health care expenditure in the developed world.[1] In the last 3 decades, the development of increasingly potent acid suppressants has revolutionized the medical management of GERD. Initially, histamine H_2-receptor antagonists (H_2-RAs) supplanted antacids for the healing of erosive esophagitis (EE); H_2-RAs were, in turn, supplanted, to a large extent, by PPIs, which provided healing and symptom relief in a significantly greater proportion of patients than H_2-RAs.[2,3] Despite the success of acid suppression, GERD is not primarily a disorder of acid secretion and there have been many attempts to develop pharmacologic, endoscopic, and surgical treatments to increase basal lower esophageal sphincter (LES) pressure, reduce the frequency and duration of inappropriate transient LES relaxations (TLESRs), improve esophageal clearance, and accelerate gastric emptying. The attractions of targeting the pathophysiologic

This article originally appeared in *Gastroenterology Clinics of North America, volume 39, 2010.*
[a] Division of Gastroenterology, HSC-4W8F, McMaster University Medical Centre, 1200 Main Street West, Hamilton, ON L8N 3Z5, Canada
[b] Barts and The London School of Medicine and Dentistry, Wingate Institute of Neurogastroenterology, 26 Ashfield Street, London E12AJ, UK
* Corresponding author.
E-mail address: d.sifrim@qmul.ac.uk

Thorac Surg Clin 21 (2011) 557–574
doi:10.1016/j.thorsurg.2011.09.005
1547-4127/11/$ – see front matter © 2011 Elsevier Inc. All rights reserved.

basis of GERD rather than acid suppression have not yielded new medications that produce healing and symptom relief comparable with those reported for PPIs.

Documented costs for managing GERD are attributable predominantly to the costs of pharmacotherapy,[4,5] although surgical therapy is also associated with substantial costs, as are over-the-counter remedies.[6-9] The costs of treating GERD and its complications have prompted close scrutiny of prescribing habits with the expectation that management guidelines and consequent constraints on pharmacotherapy will reduce expenditure.[9,10] Reports that antireflux therapy may be provided without documentation of a diagnostic indication, in up to one-third of patients,[11,12] suggest a significant opportunity to reduce the costs of GERD treatments. However, GERD is associated with an increased risk of esophageal adenocarcinoma and other complications[13,14] and with substantial impairment of patients' sleep, work productivity, and quality of life that warrant therapy.[13] Furthermore, despite apparently optimal therapy, many patients continue to experience symptoms attributable to GERD, suggesting that there are still unmet needs.

The aim of this article to is to highlight current and emerging treatments for GERD, opportunities for improving medical treatment, the extent to which improvements may be achieved with current therapy, and where new therapies may be required. These issues are discussed in the context of current thinking on the pathogenesis of GERD and its various manifestations and on the pharmacologic basis of current treatments.

PATHOPHYSIOLOGY OF GERD

The Montreal definition of GERD as "a condition which develops when the reflux of stomach contents causes troublesome symptoms and/or complications",[13] is widely accepted; however, this definition does not specify how and why reflux occurs, which organs are affected by the reflux, or what symptoms and complications may be associated with the reflux of gastric contents.

Gastroesophageal reflux (GER) occurs in healthy individuals without any obvious sequelae; it is generally considered normal for the esophagus to be exposed to gastric acid (pH <4) for up to 3% to 4% of the day (approximately 45–60 minutes a day). Similarly, TLESRs are normal events that occur in response to physiologic gastric distension. The duration of esophageal acid exposure, documented at one point, 5 cm above the LES, is often termed the reflux time; this implies that it is gastric acid or, more precisely,

esophageal luminal fluid with a pH less than 4.0, that causes GERD. However, in an unknown proportion of patients, GERD symptoms seem to be associated with the presence of weakly acidic or alkaline conditions in the esophagus, suggesting that factors other than gastric acid and pepsin may be responsible for GERD.

Thus, excessive GER can occur for several reasons (**Box 1**), which may be amenable to pharmacologic therapy; however, the range of causes is such that not all of these causes could be responsive to the same medication or to a single, standard treatment regimen. Depending on the causes of an individual's GERD, it may be appropriate to target dietary factors, motility factors, concurrent therapy, meal-related factors, daytime or night-time acid secretion, structural factors (eg, hiatal hernia), or psychological factors.

MANIFESTATIONS OF GERD

GERD is remarkable for the variety of possible causes and for its protean manifestations (**Box 2**). Although it is generally accepted that heartburn and regurgitation are diagnostic of GERD,[13] these typical symptoms may occur in the absence of GERD (so-called functional heartburn).[15] Moreover, GERD may present with other atypical symptoms referable to the esophagus or to other organs.[13] Although GER and GERD symptoms are common postprandially, recent studies highlight the association between GERD and sleep disturbances and the observation that sleep disturbances may improve with effective antireflux therapy.[13] The diurnal patterns of GER that lead to typical symptoms may therefore be different from those associated with sleep disturbance or noncardiac chest pain; similarly, the timing and duration of reflux episodes documented in patients with nonerosive reflux disease (NERD) are different from those observed in patients with EE or Barrett esophagus.[16] Data are limited with respect to the characteristics of reflux in patients with laryngopharyngitis, asthma, otitis media, or dental erosions attributed to GERD. However, it would not be surprising if, for example, the diurnal reflux patterns in patients with presumed reflux laryngopharyngitis differed from those in patients with EE. Thus, even if the causes of the reflux episodes were similar in patients with different manifestations of GER, one might expect differing therapeutic requirements for different presentations.

ACID SUPPRESSION THERAPY

For a variety of reasons, including patient adherence and commercial considerations, emphasis

Box 1
Potential mechanisms underlying symptoms or signs of GERD

Excessive GER

- Delayed gastric emptying with retention of gastric contents

  Gastroparesis

  Gastric outlet obstruction

  Small bowel dysmotility (carbohydrate, gluten intolerance)
- Hiatus hernia
- Reduced basal LES pressure
- Excessive TLESRs
- Increased gastric acid secretion

  Zollinger-Ellison syndrome

  Rebound hypersecretion after withdrawal of acid suppression therapy

  Helicobacter pylori-negative status

  Increased duodenogastroesophageal reflux

  Bile acids

  Pancreatic secretions

Excessive esophageal exposure to noxious agents

- Impaired esophageal clearance

  Disordered esophageal body motility

  Impaired salivary secretion
- Hiatus hernia
- Luminal agents

  Acidic foods

  Alcohol

  Medications (eg, bisphosphonates, antibiotics)

Excessive esophageal sensitivity

- Functional esophageal disease (Rome)
- Esophageal hyperalgesia
- Central hyperalgesia

  Depression

  Irritable bowel syndrome
- Concurrent inflammation

  Eosinophilic esophagitis

Box 2
Potential manifestations of GERD

- Symptomatic: esophageal

  Typical symptoms

     Heartburn, regurgitation

     Chest pain

     Dysphagia

  Atypical symptoms

     Abdominal pain or burning

     Nausea, vomiting
- Symptomatic: nonesophageal

  Cough

  Wheeze

  Hoarseness

  Shortness of breath

  Sleep disturbance

  Earache

  Dysphagia/globus symptoms

  Glossitis

  Toothache
- Complications

  Esophageal mucosal breaks (erosions/ulcers)

  Esophageal stricture

  Barrett esophagus

  Esophageal adenocarcinoma

  Reflux laryngopharyngitis

  Bronchitis

  Pneumonia

  Otitis media

  Dental erosions

has been placed on developing antireflux therapies that need to be taken only once daily. Although this strategy is associated with greater adherence than multiple daily doses,[17,18] it is appropriate only if the pharmacologic profile is consistent with therapeutic goals. Prompt acid neutralization by antacids is associated with rapid relief of reflux symptoms but the effect is short-lived with no prospect of antacids being used as a once-daily therapy. Histamine H_2-RAs have a significantly longer duration of action, offset by the fact that their effect is not immediate. In the treatment of GERD, H_2-RAs were evaluated twice daily; although H_2-RAs are more effective than placebo for healing EE, their long-term effectiveness is compromised by tachyphylaxis[19–23] and there is little, if any, benefit from using doses up to twice the standard healing dose.[24] The short duration of effect and tachyphylaxis of H_2-RAs limits their benefit when used once daily.

PPIs have proved significantly more effective than antacids or H_2-RAs for healing and maintaining remission in EE and for maintaining symptom relief.[2,3] Studies documented more prolonged acid suppression with PPIs than with H_2-RAs and the degree of acid suppression, because the proportion of the 24-hour period during which gastric pH exceeded 4.0 correlated with the proportion of patients with healing of their EE over 8 weeks.[25] Gastric pH studies confirmed that, although currently available PPIs have their C_{max} (maximum concentration) at 90 to 120 minutes after administration, they produce more prolonged acid suppression (gastric pH ≥ 4.0) because they are covalently bound to the proton pumps; this suppression is overcome only when new proton pumps are inserted into the secretory membrane of the parietal cell canaliculus. As a result, current PPIs, taken once daily, can produce sufficient gastric acid suppression to achieve healing and symptom relief in many patients with GERD. Despite this situation, currently available PPIs have identifiable limitations related to their mechanism of action.[26] Conventional PPIs do not have a rapid onset of action because they are prodrugs, administered in an enteric, acid-resistant formulation, to prevent premature inactivation by gastric acid; after dissolution of the enteric coating, the prodrug is absorbed in the small intestine. Because PPIs are weak bases, they are concentrated in the highly acidic, secretory canaliculus; activation of the prodrug to its sulphenamide form occurs only in the acidic secretory canaliculus of an actively secreting parietal cell, when the activated sulphenamide produces irreversible inhibition of those proton pumps (H^+-K^+ ATPase) that are actively inserted in the secretory canalicular membrane. These events occur only if circulating blood levels are high enough to allow sufficient PPI prodrug to concentrate in active parietal cells; however, because conventional PPIs have a t_{max} (time of maximum concentration) of about 1 to 6 hours and a half-life of about 60 to 130 minutes, the PPI plasma residence time is less than 12 hours (**Fig. 1**), such that plasma levels decrease below the therapeutic threshold within 4 to 10 hours of drug ingestion.[27,28] Parietal cells that become active more than 4 to 10 hours after drug ingestion remain uninhibited because plasma PPI levels have fallen below the therapeutic threshold (**Fig. 2**); as a result, gastric acidity steadily recovers over the 16 to 18 hours that remain until the next single daily dose. Because blocked proton pumps are not replaced for 3 to 4 days, PPIs have a progressively greater effect in reducing gastric acidity over the first 3 to 5 days

of administration but, despite this, their effect diminishes over the 24-hour period between doses as new proton pumps are synthesized and acid secretion gradually increases.[29] This situation may not be a problem for many patients with GERD whose symptoms occur predominantly during the daytime but, for other patients, the loss of PPI effect may permit nocturnal return of acid secretion (**Fig. 3**A) and nocturnal acid reflux (see **Fig. 3**B), leading to persistent night-time symptoms on once-daily PPI therapy. For some patients, the PPI effect is influenced by differences in PPI pharmacokinetics; variability in blood PPI levels, and hence in gastric acidity, and may be to the result of differences in absorption or differences in PPI metabolism related, for example, to CYP2C19 polymorphisms.[30,31] As a result, 24-hour gastric acidity can vary by as much as 3 to 4 log units between individuals (**Fig. 4**); furthermore, this interindividual variability does not seem to disappear after 3 days of once-daily oral dosing.[32]

Pure PPI isomers, such as esomeprazole, dexlansoprazole, and TU-199 (an isomer of tenatoprazole), generally produce higher blood levels than the racemic mixtures, leading to an increase in gastric acid suppression; in early studies with esomeprazole, the increase in gastric acid suppression was attributed to an increased area under the curve (AUC) for the concentration-time curve[33,34] but more recent studies with dexlansoprazole[35] and other PPIs suggest that there is a threshold effect; that is, regardless of the peak concentration or AUC, acid suppression is achieved as long as blood levels exceed a threshold level.[35–37] In clinical practice, threshold blood levels can be maintained by multiple daily oral dosing[38,39] or by continuous infusion as in the management of upper gastrointestinal bleeding.[39–41] Multiple daily dosing regimens raise concerns about patient adherence, and concerns remain that first-generation PPIs are slow to achieve an effective reduction in gastric acidity.

Recognition that current PPIs do not address all clinical needs has led to new antisecretory agents that offer more rapid onset and a more prolonged duration of action.[42,43] Speed of onset has been addressed by an immediate-release (IR) omeprazole formulation that contains uncoated omeprazole powder (20 mg or 40 mg) plus sodium bicarbonate (1680 mg)[44]; the sodium bicarbonate neutralizes gastric acid, protecting the acid-labile omeprazole from degradation and, in addition, stimulating gastrin release by increasing gastric pH; the latter effect stimulates insertion of acid pumps, analogous to food-stimulated acid secretion, such that the parietal cells are activated

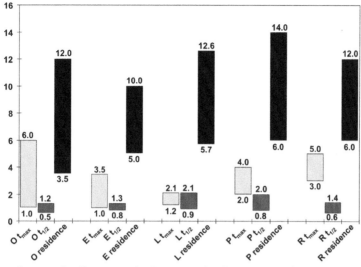

Omeprazole Esomeprazole Lansoprazole Pantoprazole Rabeprazole

Fig. 1. Pharmacokinetic data for 5 PPIs that are widely available; t_{max} and $t_{1/2}$ vary for each drug, with t_{max} ranging overall from 1.0 hours to 6.0 hours and $t_{1/2}$ ranging overall from 0.5 hours to 3.5 hours; the calculated residence time (the time, after ingestion, during which the plasma concentrations remain greater than 3% of the C_{max}) does not exceed 14.0 hours for any PPI. (*Data from* Klotz U. Pharmacokinetic considerations in the eradication of *Helicobacter pylori*. Clin Pharmacokinet 2000;38:243–70; and Shi S, Klotz U. Proton pump inhibitors: an update of their clinical use and pharmacokinetics. Eur J Clin Pharmacol 2008;64:935–51.)

and, hence, susceptible to omeprazole. The antisecretory effect of IR omeprazole is evident more quickly than that of classic delayed-release PPIs.[45–47] Esomeprazole, the first pure isomer PPI, produces a greater AUC than racemic omeprazole, and the associated increase in acid

suppression is associated with a small, but significant increase in healing rates for EE.[48–53] Another approach to prolonged acid suppression is to extend the period during which blood levels of the PPI exceed the threshold level needed to achieve therapeutic levels of the PPI in the

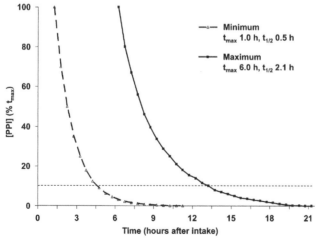

Fig. 2. Simulated plasma concentration curves for 2 theoretic PPIs that have the shortest t_{max} and $t_{1/2}$ (minimum) and longest t_{max} and $t_{1/2}$ (maximum) reported for the 5 PPIs that are, currently, most widely available; even under the latter conditions (maximum), plasma concentrations decrease to less than 10% off the C_{max} by 13 to 14 hours after PPI ingestion. Thus, minimal PPI is available to inhibit proton pump function for the last 8 to 11 hours of the day in patients receiving once-daily PPI. (*Data from* Klotz U. Pharmacokinetic considerations in the eradication of *Helicobacter pylori*. Clin Pharmacokinet 2000;38:243–70; and Shi S, Klotz U. Proton pump inhibitors: an update of their clinical use and pharmacokinetics. Eur J Clin Pharmacol 2008;64:935–51.)

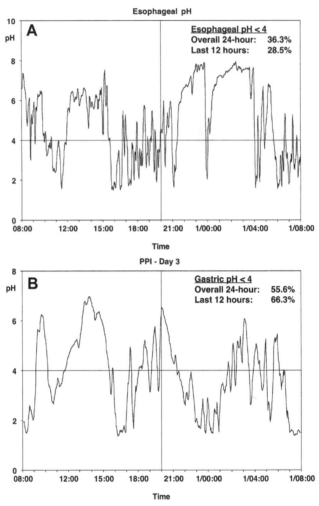

Fig. 3. Luminal pH recordings from (*A*) the esophagus and (*B*) the stomach. (*A*) A 24-hour esophageal pH recording, off therapy, from a patient who has severe LA grade C EE; there is significant esophageal acid exposure through the day but, importantly, there is prolonged acid exposure during the latter half of the recording (pH < 4.0 for 28.5% of the recording). (*B*) A 24-hour gastric pH recording in a healthy, *H pylori*-negative patient after 3 days of rabeprazole, 20 mg daily; during the latter half of the recording, the gastric pH is acidic (<4.0) for 66.3% of the time.

secretory canaliculus of the parietal cell. Dexlansoprazole, the R-isomer of lansoprazole, is metabolized more slowly than the S-isomer; it is now approved in the United States as a modified, dual-release formulation in which some of the R-isomer has a standard enteric coating and some a modified coating that releases the PPI at a higher pH; as a result, there is a second peak in blood levels and a more prolonged increase of dexlansoprazole levels above threshold levels. Clinically, dual-release dexlansoprazole (60 mg and 90 mg daily) healed EE after 8 weeks in 92.7% and 93.3% of patients, respectively, whereas standard lansoprazole, 30 mg daily, produced healing in 88.9% of patients (*P*<.01).[54] Although differences for healing, symptom relief, and maintenance of

remission[55–57] are comparable with the differences between esomeprazole 40 mg daily and omeprazole 20 mg daily,[49,50] it is not clear how much of the effect is because of the change in formulation and how much to the absolute increase in dosage. Neither of the other isomeric PPIs, S-pantoprazole[58] or dexrabeprazole,[59] is available clinically and their benefit in clinical practice remains uncertain.[60]

Other PPIs, still in development, include AGN 201,904-Z,[37] ilaprazole (IY-81,149),[61] and tenatoprazole (TU-199).[36,62–66] AGN 201,904-Z, the sodium salt of an acid stable omeprazole prodrug, is designed to provide continued metered absorption throughout the gut and, thus, prolong the plasma PPI residence time; the prodrug is

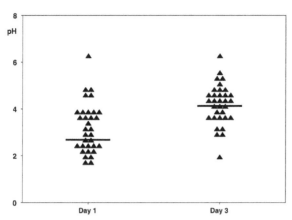

Fig. 4. Median 24-hour gastric pH values from 33 healthy, *H pylori*-negative patients on the first (day 1) and third (day 3) days during which they received rabeprazole 20 mg daily. The group median pH values were 3.1 (day 1) and 4.3 (day 3) but there was marked, interpatient variability with respect to the individual median 24-hour gastric pH values. (*Data from* Armstrong D, James C, Camacho F, et al. Oral rabeprazole vs. intravenous pantoprazole: a comparison of the effect on intragastric pH in healthy subjects. Aliment Pharmacol Ther 2007;25:185–96.)

converted rapidly to omeprazole in the systemic circulation, producing faster and greater acid suppression than esomeprazole 40 mg daily in healthy, *H pylori*-negative male volunteers.[37] Ilaprazole is a benzimidazole derivative that has a longer half-life and greater acid suppression than omeprazole.[42] Racemic tenatoprazole, an imidazopyridine derivative, has a longer half-life ($t_{1/2} \sim$ 8–9 hours) than first-generation benzimidazole-derived PPIs, with the result that it produces a significantly higher median 24-hour pH than esomeprazole, 40 mg daily, after 7 days' administration.[62–64] A crossover study comparing isomeric S-tenatoprazole sodium, 30 mg, 60 mg, and 90 mg daily, with esomeprazole, 40 mg daily, showed that the higher doses produced significantly greater and more prolonged dose-dependent 24-hour and nocturnal acid suppression than esomeprazole.[66] A meta-analysis of individual subject data from 4 pharmacodynamic studies has shown, also, that S-tenatoprazole sodium, 60 mg daily, produces greater acid suppression than esomeprazole, 40 mg daily, and is comparable with esomeprazole, 40 mg twice daily,[67] although there are no clinical trial data in patients.

In the last few years, another class of acid suppressants has been developed; the P-CABs also inhibit the H^+-K^+ ATPase but, unlike PPIs, they target the potassium-binding region of the proton pump. P-CABs are lipophilic weak bases with a high pKa and are stable at low pH. They are absorbed rapidly and are concentrated, up to 100,000-fold, in the secretory canaliculus; the protonated form then binds ionically, but reversibly to the proton pump,[68] producing rapid and profound acid suppression.[69,70] Initial studies with

P-CABs such as linaprazan (AZD-0865), revaprazan (YH1885), and soraprazan indicated that these compounds have a more rapid onset of action and the potential for greater acid suppression than conventional PPIs.[71–74] Linaprazan (AZD-0865) given once daily was not superior to esomeprazole, 40 mg daily, in the treatment of EE and NERD,[75,76] and the development program for this compound has been halted.

Although antacids and H_2-RAs are less effective than PPIs, they still have a role in management of patients with GERD, particularly as over-the-counter medications.[77] As prescription medications, H_2-RAs alone are not, generally, effective for more severe grades of GERD; however, they are still recommended and used widely for patients with mild or infrequent symptoms[78,79] and also, in combination with PPIs, for patients with persistent nocturnal symptoms.[80] Initial enthusiasm for combined therapy with a PPI and an H_2-RA[81] was tempered by a diminution in benefit that was observed as tachyphylaxis to the H_2-RA developed[19,82]; however, more recent data, and studies with combinations of a PPI and an H_2-RA, suggest that there is still a role for combination acid suppression therapy in some patients with GERD.[42,79–81,83]

NONACID SUPPRESSION THERAPY

Acid suppression therapy remains the mainstay of medical management for GERD, and PPIs provide the most effective acid suppression therapy. Despite this, PPIs are less effective for complete symptom relief and, furthermore, relapse of symptoms and complications such as erosions, strictures, and hemorrhage can occur, even with maintenance PPI therapy. There are good pharmacologic reasons why some patients might not respond to standard, once-daily therapy with a PPI and, although there is good reason to assume that increased acid suppression improves response rates, there are several other mechanisms that might underlie PPI failure in GERD, including the presence of esophagitis or other esophageal diseases, persistent weakly acidic reflux or duodenogastroesophageal reflux, delayed gastric emptying, esophageal hypersensitivity, concomitant functional bowel disorders, and psychological comorbidity. Identification of the individual underlying mechanisms for persistent symptoms, where possible, might be relevant for the management of refractory GERD. Several agents under development may have a role in selected refractory reflux patients. They include motility agents to accelerate gastric emptying and improve esophageal clearance, antireflux agents that reduce the frequency of TLESRs and thereby the number of acid and nonacid reflux episodes, visceral pain modulators to reduce visceral hypersensitivity, and mucosal protection agents. None of these agents, on its own, is likely to be as effective as a PPI in so many patients but there may be a role for these medications in combination with acid suppression therapy.

MOTILITY AGENTS

A significant factor in the pathophysiology of GERD is disordered gastroesophageal motility,[84] including one or more of these abnormalities: delayed gastric emptying, reduced LES pressure, increased incidence of reflux during TLESRs, and ineffective esophageal clearance. Together with a hiatal hernia, disordered gastroesophageal motility may favor GER and/or determine the volume, proximal extent, and composition of the refluxates. Gastroesophageal hypomotility might be a cofactor involved in refractoriness to PPI treatment.[85] Several prokinetic agents can stimulate gastrointestinal motility and many of these agents have been used, either alone or in combination with a PPI or H_2-RA, for the treatment of GERD. Bethanechol, metoclopramide, domperidone, cisapride, and macrolides, such as erythromycin or ABT-229, have all been used in patients with GERD.[86–97] Although these drugs are believed predominantly to impart their effect by enhancing esophageal motility, reflux clearance, basal LES pressure, reducing TLESRs, and by accelerating gastric emptying, many of these compounds are not highly selective and have off-target effects. This situation means that the mechanism of action responsible for their therapeutic effects often remains controversial, and undesirable side effects are often encountered. For example, cisapride, a $5-HT_4$ agonist that was approved for use in GERD before subsequently being withdrawn for safety reasons, not only increased the rate of gastric emptying but also modified saliva secretion and bicarbonate content and gastric acid secretion, believed to occur via potassium channels,[92,98] which also mediated the adverse cardiac effects of cisapride. Although cisapride was more effective than placebo in symptom relief and healing esophagitis, studies indicated that cisapride has little effect on esophageal motility and, notably, no effect on TLESRs after 4 weeks of oral (20 mg twice daily) administration.[89] Tegaserod, another partially selective $5-HT_4$ agonist, also showed some efficacy in small GERD trials. Tegaserod (1 and 4 mg/d) reduced postprandial reflux and TLESRs but did not alter LES tone.[93] However, as with cisapride, it is uncertain whether the beneficial effects of tegaserod were because of the effect on motor function or other recently documented effects on salivary flow rate, salivary bicarbonate and epidermal growth factor secretion, and bicarbonate secretion from esophageal submucosal glands.[99,100] Tegaserod has also been withdrawn from the market for safety issues.

Motilin is a peptide found in specific endocrine cells in the epithelia of the upper small intestine.[101,102] Motilin receptor agonists can increase gastric emptying after ingestion of a meal; this action is mediated via the cholinergic system of the stomach.[103] Much of this evidence is derived from the use of erythromycin, a macrolide antibiotic that also acts as a motilin receptor agonist.[95] Erythromycin, given at low doses, which have no antibiotic effect, was the first motilin agonist used in several clinical situations, particularly in severe gastroparesis. Early studies found erythromycin to be of no value in the control of reflux.[86] ABT-229, an erythromycin derivative devoid of antibiotic activity, accelerates gastric emptying and increases LES pressure[103] in healthy persons; however, the therapeutic effect of ABT-229 in patients with GERD was limited in terms of modulation of both esophageal motility (LES pressure and TLESRs) and acid exposure.[104,105] The development of ABT-229 has been discontinued because of a rapid onset of tachyphylaxis and worsening of symptoms in dyspeptic patients. In a recent study in patients after lung transplantation, another macrolide antibiotic, azithromycin, reduced the number of reflux events and total esophageal acid exposure and also reduced the proximal extent to which reflux regurgitated.[94]

There are several limitations when using macrolides as prokinetics in GERD. The most consistent data supporting their role as prokinetics in reflux disease come from studies in which the drug was administered intravenously[86,88,106]; this would not be suitable for a broader GERD population. In addition, repeat administration of macrolides induces desensitization of the motilin receptor, reducing their efficacy over time.[102,107] Macrolides also induce side effects, including nausea and abdominal cramping, which are believed to be caused by direct activation of motilin receptors on gastric smooth muscle, which occurs at higher doses[102] and which makes macrolides difficult to tolerate for many patients. A more selective motilin agonist, which could be taken orally, would be highly desirable to test in patients with GERD with compromised gastroesophageal motor function.

Few studies have assessed the value of the current therapeutic approach to delayed gastric emptying in patients with GERD, who failed PPI therapy. However, it is likely that these patients also complain about other dyspeptic symptoms related to slow gastric motor activity. There are no data about the value of adding a promotility drug in patients who have failed PPI therapy, given once or twice per day. However, in patients with delayed gastric emptying and persistent GERD symptoms on PPI therapy, the use of a promotility agent remains an attractive option.

ANTIREFLUX AGENTS

Prevention of GER, either acidic or nonacidic, should be the ultimate goal of GERD treatment. As reflux mainly occurs during TLESRs,[108,109] drugs targeting this motor pattern may be useful to reduce GERD symptoms.[110,111] Although most studies show no difference in the number of TLESRs, between healthy individuals and patients with GERD, patients with GERD have acid reflux twice as often during a TLESR compared with healthy individuals.[112,113] A recent study described a possible reason for this difference. The position of a proximal gastric acid pocket is largely determined by the presence of a hiatal hernia. Entrapment of the pocket above the diaphragm, especially in patients with hiatal hernia, is a major risk factor underlying the increased occurrence of acidic reflux during a TLESR in patients with GERD.[114] The importance of hiatal hernia and other reflux mechanisms, such as straining, absent LES pressure, and reflux induced by swallowing, should also be emphasized when considering the efficacy of drugs aimed at reducing the occurrence of TLESRs.

Several pharmacologic agents, including γ-aminobutyric acid-B (GABA$_B$[115–123]) and GABA$_A$ receptor agonists,[124] cholecystokinin A antagonists,[125] morphine,[126] glutamate antagonists,[127] cannabinoids,[128,129] metabotropic glutamate receptor agonists and antagonists,[129–131] and nitric oxide synthase inhibitors,[132] all reduce the triggering of TLESRs. These drugs have not reached clinical development, mainly owing to their undesirable pharmacologic profile and/or side effects.

GABA$_B$ RECEPTOR AGONISTS

Baclofen, a GABA$_B$ receptor agonist, used in the clinical management of spasticity, reduces TLESRs in animals[133] and healthy volunteers.[118] The maximal inhibition of TLESRs provoked by baclofen in humans varies between 40% and 60%.[118,121] Administration of baclofen also increases basal LES pressure and reduces the number of reflux episodes in patients with GERD.[115–117,119–121,134] One study evaluated the effect of baclofen (4–10 mg daily) for 4 weeks in patients with GERD[116] and showed a significant reduction in acid exposure and symptoms. These results reinforce the point that reflux inhibition is a valid concept in treating GERD, because the inhibition of TLESRs seems to be associated with a reduction in acid exposure. Furthermore, they show that humans do not become tolerant of baclofen when it is taken for a longer period. Short-term studies showed that baclofen was also effective in patients with hiatal hernia.[135] However, because baclofen increases basal LES pressure it is possible that this effect adds to the effect on TLESRs in patients with hiatal hernia.

Baclofen not only reduces acid reflux but also has a similar inhibitory effect on nonacid reflux and duodenal reflux. Vela and colleagues[120] showed that 40 mg of baclofen reduced both postprandial acid and nonacid reflux measured with impedance-pH monitoring and decreased associated symptoms in healthy individuals and patients with heartburn. Similarly, Koek and colleagues[117] showed that baclofen (5 mg, 3 times daily) effectively reduced duodenal reflux (measured by Bilitec) and associated PPI-resistant symptoms.

Arbaclofen placarbil is a prodrug of R-baclofen, the active stereoisomer of baclofen. A recent trial in 50 patients with GERD revealed that it is well tolerated and reduced the number of reflux episodes and associated heartburn.[136] However, the effect was marginal and larger studies are required.

Baclofen has effects on the central nervous system (CNS) that limit its value for treating GERD. As the drug crosses the blood-brain barrier, a variety of CNS-related side effects may occur, including somnolence, confusion, dizziness, lightheadedness, drowsiness, weakness, and trembling. Baclofen has a short pharmacologic half-life (3–4 hours), which necessitates dosing 3 or more times per day.

Attention is focusing on the development of new GABA$_B$ receptor agonists that act primarily at peripheral sites and therefore have better tolerability. For example, lesogaberan[137] has a similar pharmacodynamic effect on reflux parameters to baclofen, resulting in almost complete inhibition of TLESRs in dogs, and a similar degree of inhibition as baclofen in healthy individuals.[122] However, in contrast to baclofen, this agent seems to act in the periphery, with a low incidence of CNS-related adverse effects, making it more interesting as an add-on therapy for the treatment of patients with GERD with an incomplete response to PPI therapy. A recent randomized trial with 232 patients has shown a significant difference in symptom response with lesogaberan compared with placebo.[138]

GLUTAMATE RECEPTOR ANTAGONISTS

Glutamate is involved in the vagovagal reflex, triggering TLESRs. Glutamate binds to metabotropic glutamate receptors (mGluRs) structurally related to GABA$_B$ receptors. A recent study showed that riluzole (a benzothiazole inhibiting the release of excitatory amino acids such as glutamate and aspartate) attenuated the rate of TLESRs triggered by isovolumetric distention in healthy volunteers.[127]

More selective mGluR5 antagonists potently inhibit TLESRs and reflux in ferrets and dogs.[130,139] Recent studies showed that ADX10059, a potent, selective, negative allosteric modulator of mGluR5, improved esophageal pH-metry and clinical symptoms in patients with GERD.[131,140] Further development of this drug for chronic use in reflux disease was canceled because of liver toxicity.

CANNABINOID RECEPTOR AGONISTS

Cannabinoid CB$_1$ receptors have been localized in brain areas involved in the triggering of TLESRs. A study in dogs showed that the CB receptor agonist WIN 55,212-2 reduced the occurrence of TLESRs in response to gastric distension by 80%.[128] A study in ferrets confirmed involvement of CB$_1$ receptors in the central regulation of LES relaxation and showed the presence of CB$_1$ receptors in the brain centers involved in the triggering of TLESRs.[141] These data indicate that CB$_1$ agonists may be clinically useful to reduce TLESRs in

humans but, like baclofen, central side effects were reported and so more specific CB$_1$ agonists devoid of central side effects need to be further investigated.

PPI treatment does not abolish nonacid reflux[142] and the esophagus continues to be exposed to gastric contents with mild ongoing mucosal irritation and possible persistence of symptoms. Patients with GERD who failed PPI therapy may show an association between their symptoms and 3 different types of GER: weak acidic/alkaline reflux, acidic reflux, and duodenal GER. Drugs targeting the mechanisms underlying GER or TLESRs could also reduce nonacid and DGER. Patients with NERD or low-grade esophagitis mainly reflux during TLESRs. This subgroup should benefit most from drugs that reduce TLESRs. More probably, the best indication for reflux inhibitors in GERD is to improve PPI-resistant symptoms by reducing persistent nonacid and acid reflux. This strategy implies that reflux inhibitors are prescribed as add-on treatment in this subgroup of patients.

VISCERAL PAIN MODULATORS

There are no studies specifically evaluating the value of visceral pain modulators in patients with GERD with persistent heartburn despite PPI treatment. However, given that most patients who fail PPI treatment originate from the NERD group, and that up to 40% of PPI failures show a lack of either weak or acidic reflux during intraesophageal impedance assessment, the use of these agents is highly attractive. Pain modulators such as tricyclic antidepressants, trazodone, and selective serotonin reuptake inhibitors (SSRIs) all improve esophageal pain in patients with noncardiac chest pain.[143–145] It is thought that these agents confer their visceral analgesic effect by acting on the CNS and/or sensory afferents. The pain modulators are used in nonmood-altering doses, and provide a therapeutic alternative until more novel and esophageal-specific compounds become available.

Human studies supporting a spinal mechanism in the development of visceral hypersensitivity are limited; however, using a model of acid-induced esophageal pain hypersensitivity, the development of secondary allodynia in the nonacid-exposed proximal esophagus after a distal esophageal acid infusion has been shown.[146] This secondary allodynia is believed to occur through sensitization of spinal neurons, and can be attenuated by both the prostaglandin E$_2$ receptor-1[147] and N-methyl-D-aspartate receptor antagonist, ketamine.[148] These studies suggest that spinal neurons can induce visceral hypersensitivity and may also be treated using specific therapies.

MUCOSAL PROTECTION

The human esophagus contains esophageal submucosal glands (SMGs), which secrete bicarbonate, mucin, and other products. Esophageal SMG secretions are likely to serve a protective effect against injury to the mucosa by refluxed gastric acid either by direct buffering of luminal acid or by creating a preepithelial defense and buffer zone close to the mucosal surface. Given these observations, drugs that stimulate SMG secretion may have beneficial effects in patients with GERD.

Sucralfate is protective against acid or acid-pepsin injury to rabbit and cat esophagus. Its beneficial action is due, in part, to enhanced mucosal defense (cytoprotection) because it can occur in the absence of luminal buffering of hydrogen ion.[149]

Tegaserod is a secretogogue that increases duodenal bicarbonate secretion; the presence of serotonin receptors in the esophagus may explain the finding that tegaserod stimulates esophageal SMG bicarbonate secretion, an effect that likely accounts for the observed protection against acid-pepsin injury to pig, but not rabbit, esophagus.[99]

Exposure of esophageal epithelial cells to unconjugated bile acids increases intracellular reactive oxygen species, and this effect is blocked by antioxidants. Recent preliminary studies showed that changes in esophageal mucosal integrity induced by weakly acidic solutions with unconjugated bile acids, similar to reflux in patients with GERD on PPI, can be prevented with antioxidants.[150]

IMPLICATIONS FOR CURRENT CLINICAL PRACTICE

Current PPIs, given once daily, achieve healing in more than 90% of patients with mild EE (Los Angeles [LA] grade A).[2,48-52] Although healing rates are markedly lower for more severe EE (LA grades C and D),[53] and 6-month remission rates on maintenance therapy are generally less than 75% to 85%,[151,152] it has been proposed that increased acid suppression produces little improvement in outcomes.[153,154] This proposition, along with reports linking acid suppression therapy to gastrointestinal infections, fractures, vitamin B_{12} deficiency and respiratory infections,[1,43] has triggered considerable interest in alternative antireflux therapies to address the substantial impairment in quality of life and a risk of complications associated with GERD.[14,155]

However, there is no direct alternative to PPI therapy. Although GERD symptoms may persist, despite healing of EE,[49-52] in up to 40% of patients with GERD taking once-daily PPI therapy,[131,153,154,156] there are no data to indicate that other agents are more effective for healing or symptom resolution. Similarly, persistent symptoms in patients diagnosed with NERD may indicate that they have functional heartburn rather than true GERD[157,158] but, in most trials, patients with NERD have received lower-dose PPIs for a shorter period than EE patients and there are no data to indicate that other agents would be more effective. Complete absence of a response to once-daily PPI therapy may suggest PPI failure[154,159] but an incomplete response does not necessarily indicate PPI failure.[154] There are few clinical data on multiple daily dosing for current PPIs despite the fact that once-daily dosing does not produce maximal acid suppression,[160] that twice-daily dosing produces greater acid suppression,[38] and that multiple daily doses or a continuous infusion may be required for upper gastrointestinal hemorrhage[39-41,161] or Zollinger-Ellison syndrome.[162] Under these circumstances, it is reasonable to consider a trial of more effective acid suppression for patients who have persistent symptoms when taking a PPI once daily.

The pharmacology of current, first-generation PPIs mitigates against day-long acid suppression or a rapid onset of action. Thus, persistent GERD symptoms and complications in patients receiving once-daily PPI therapy may respond to more prolonged acid suppression regimens, for example, with multiple daily dosing of a current PPI or single daily dosing of a new PPI that has a longer plasma residence time. Similarly, ineffective on-demand therapy may respond to IR PPIs. If increased acid suppression is ineffective, persistent symptoms may then indicate the need to address other mechanisms with, for example, prokinetics, antireflux medications, visceral sensory modulators, or mucosal protectants (**Box 3**). Based on studies to date, these agents should probably be considered as supplements to PPI therapy, tailored to the patient's symptom and disease profile and to the pharmacologic profile of the drugs.

IMPLICATIONS FOR THE FUTURE

The management of severe or persistent GERD[51-53,151,152] and its complications is likely to benefit from acid suppression agents that have a longer half-life and plasma residence time, leading to more prolonged acid suppression.

Box 3
Therapeutic options for persistent GERD symptoms

- Optimization of once-daily PPI therapy

  Ensure adherence

  Take before breakfast

  Switch to different PPI

    PPI with slower metabolism

    Pure isomeric PPI

    IR PPI for rapid onset

  Modify diet: avoid foods that delay gastric emptying or promote reflux

- Supplementation of once-daily PPI therapy

  Antacids for acute, infrequent exacerbations

    Intermittent

  Bicarbonate, with PPI, to accelerate PPI absorption

  H_2-RA therapy (nocturnal)

    Intermittent

  Prokinetic therapy

    Domperidone

    Metoclopramide

  Reflux inhibitory therapy

    Baclofen

  Epithelial protection

    Sulcrate

- Increase of PPI therapy

  Twice-daily therapy

  Multiple daily dose therapy

- Use of sensory modulator (with or without acid suppression)

  Tricyclic antidepressant

  SSRI antidepressant therapy

  Antispasmodic for reflux-induced spasm

    Nitrates

    Anticholinergic

    Botulinal toxin (endoscopic)

The management of persistent and, possibly, extraesophageal GERD symptoms requires more sophisticated measurement tools for patient-reported outcomes to provide objective documentation of symptoms and their response to therapy in individual patients.[157,158,163,164] There will then be opportunities for additional pharmacologic therapies to address gastrointestinal sensorimotor dysfunction and also for more refined treatment strategies. Contrary to common perceptions, GERD remains an enigmatic condition, the management of which continues to challenge patients and physicians alike.

REFERENCES

1. Hanauer SB. Addicted to acid suppression. Nat Rev Gastroenterol Hepatol 2009;6:497.
2. Chiba N, De Gara CJ, Wilkinson JM, et al. Speed of healing and symptom relief in grade II to IV gastro-esophageal reflux disease: a meta-analysis. Gastroenterology 1997;112(6):1798–810.
3. van Pinxteren B, Sigterman KE, Bonis P, et al. Short-term treatment with proton pump inhibitors, H2-receptor antagonists and prokinetics for gastro-oesophageal reflux disease-like symptoms and endoscopy negative reflux disease. Cochrane Database Syst Rev 2006;3:CD002095.
4. Everhart JE, Ruhl CE. Burden of digestive diseases in the United States part I: overall and upper gastrointestinal diseases. Gastroenterology 2009; 136:376–86.
5. Shaheen NJ. The burden of gastrointestinal and liver diseases, 2006. Am J Gastroenterol 2006; 101:2128–38.
6. Sonnenberg A. Motion-Laparoscopic Nissen fundoplication is more cost effective than oral PPI administration: arguments against the motion. Can J Gastroenterol 2002;16:627–31.
7. Swanstrom LL. Motion-Laparoscopic Nissen fundoplication is more cost effective than oral PPI administration: arguments for the motion. Can J Gastroenterol 2002;16:621–3.
8. Heikkinen TJ, Haukipuro K, Koivukangas P, et al. Comparison of costs between laparoscopic and open Nissen fundoplication: a prospective randomized study with a 3-month followup. J Am Coll Surg 1999;188:368–76.
9. Gerson LB, Robbins AS, Garber A, et al. A cost-effectiveness analysis of prescribing strategies in the management of gastroesophageal reflux disease. Am J Gastroenterol 2000;95:395–407.
10. Heidelbaugh JJ, Goldberg KL, Inadomi JM. Over-utilization of proton pump inhibitors: a review of cost-effectiveness and risk. Am J Gastroenterol 2009;104:S27–32.
11. Reimer C, Sondergaard B, Hilsted L, et al. Proton-pump inhibitor therapy induces acid-related symptoms in healthy volunteers after withdrawal of therapy. Gastroenterology 2009;137:80–7.
12. McColl KE, Gillen D. Evidence that proton-pump inhibitor therapy induces the symptoms it is used to treat. Gastroenterology 2009;137:20–2.

13. Vakil N, van Zanten SV, Kahrilas P, et al. The Montreal definition and classification of gastroesophageal reflux disease: a global evidence-based consensus. Am J Gastroenterol 2006;101:1900–20.

14. Lagergren J, Bergström R, Lindgren A, et al. Symptomatic gastroesophageal reflux as a risk factor for esophageal adenocarcinoma. N Engl J Med 1999; 340:825–31.

15. Clouse RE, Richter JE, Heading RC, et al. Functional esophageal disorders. Gut 1999;45(Suppl II): II31–6.

16. Dickman R, Bautista JM, Wong WM, et al. Comparison of esophageal acid exposure distribution along the esophagus among the different gastroesophageal reflux disease (GERD) groups. Am J Gastroenterol 2006;101:2463–9.

17. Gosselin A, Luo R, Lohoues H, et al. The impact of proton pump inhibitor compliance on health-care resource utilization and costs in patients with gastroesophageal reflux disease. Value Health 2009;12:34–9.

18. Tindall W. New approaches to adherence issues when dosing oral aminosalicylates in ulcerative colitis. Am J Health Syst Pharm 2009;66:451–7.

19. Fackler WK, Ours TM, Vaezi MF, et al. Long-term effect of H_2-RA therapy on nocturnal gastric acid breakthrough. Gastroenterology 2002;122:625–32.

20. Wilder-Smith CH, Halter F, Merki HS. Tolerance and rebound to H_2-receptor antagonists: intragastric acidity in patients with duodenal ulcer. Dig Dis Sci 1991;36:1685–90.

21. Lachman L, Howden CW. Twenty-four-hour intragastric pH: tolerance within 5 days of continuous ranitidine administration. Am J Gastroenterol 2000;95:57–61.

22. Wilder-Smith C, Halter F, Ernest T, et al. Loss of acid suppression during dosing with H_2-receptor antagonists. Aliment Pharmacol Ther 1990; 4(Suppl 1):15–27.

23. Nwokolo CU, Prewett EJ, Sawyerr AF, et al. Tolerance during 5 months of dosing with ranitidine, 150 mg nightly: a placebo-controlled, double-blind study. Gastroenterology 1991;101:948–53.

24. Kahrilas PJ, Fennerty MB, Joelsson B. High- versus standard-dose ranitidine for control of heartburn in poorly responsive acid reflux disease: a prospective, controlled trial. Am J Gastroenterol 1999;94:92–7.

25. Bell NJ, Burget D, Howden CW, et al. Appropriate acid suppression for the management of gastrooesophageal reflux disease. Digestion 1992;51(Suppl 1): 59–67.

26. Sachs G, Shin JM, Howden CW. Review article: the clinical pharmacology of proton pump inhibitors. Aliment Pharmacol Ther 2006;23(Suppl 2):2–8.

27. Klotz U. Pharmacokinetic considerations in the eradication of *Helicobacter pylori*. Clin Pharm 2000;38:243–70.

28. Shi S, Klotz U. Proton pump inhibitors: an update of their clinical use and pharmacokinetics. Eur J Clin Pharmacol 2008;64:935–51.

29. Shin JM, Sachs G. Pharmacology of proton pump inhibitors. Curr Gastroenterol Rep 2008;10:528–34.

30. Klotz U. Clinical impact of CYP2C19 polymorphism on the action of proton pump inhibitors: a review of a special problem. Int J Clin Pharmacol Ther 2006; 44:297–302.

31. Saitoh T, Otsuka H, Kawasaki T, et al. Influences of CYP2C19 polymorphism on recurrence of reflux esophagitis during proton pump inhibitor maintenance therapy. Hepatogastroenterology 2009;56: 703–6.

32. Armstrong D, James C, Camacho F, et al. Oral rabeprazole vs. intravenous pantoprazole: a comparison of the effect on intragastric pH in healthy subjects. Aliment Pharmacol Ther 2007;25:185–96.

33. Junghard O, Hassan-Alin M, Hasselgren G. The effect of the area under the plasma concentration vs time curve and the maximum plasma concentration of esomeprazole on intragastric pH. Eur J Clin Pharmacol 2002;58:453–8.

34. Hassan-Alin M, Andersson T, Niazi M, et al. A pharmacokinetic study comparing single and repeated oral doses of 20 mg and 40 mg omeprazole and its two optical isomers, S-omeprazole (esomeprazole) and R-omeprazole, in healthy subjects. Eur J Clin Pharmacol 2005;60:779–84.

35. Aslam N, Wright R. Dexlansoprazole MR. Expert Opin Pharmacother 2009;10:2329–36.

36. Shin JM, Homerin M, Domagala F, et al. Characterization of the inhibitory activity of tenatoprazole on the gastric H^+, K^+-ATPase in vitro and in vivo. Biochem Pharmacol 2006;71:837–49.

37. Hunt RH, Armstrong D, Yaghoobi M, et al. Predictable, prolonged suppression of gastric acidity with a novel proton pump inhibitor, AGN 201904-Z. Aliment Pharmacol Ther 2008;28:187–97.

38. Katz PO, Castell DO, Chen Y, et al. Intragastric acid suppression and pharmacokinetics of twice-daily esomeprazole: a randomized, three-way crossover study. Aliment Pharmacol Ther 2004; 20:399–406.

39. Laine L, Shah A, Bemanian S. Intragastric pH with oral vs intravenous bolus plus infusion proton-pump inhibitor therapy in patients with bleeding ulcers. Gastroenterology 2008;134:1836–41.

40. Lau JY, Sung JJ, Lee KK, et al. Effect of intravenous omeprazole on recurrent bleeding after endoscopic treatment of bleeding peptic ulcers. N Engl J Med 2000;343:310–6.

41. Sung JJ, Chan FK, Lau JY, et al. The effect of endoscopic therapy in patients receiving omeprazole for bleeding ulcers with nonbleeding visible vessels or adherent clots. A randomized comparison. Ann Intern Med 2003;139:237–43.

42. Scarpignato C, Hunt RH. Proton pump inhibitors: the beginning of the end or the end of the beginning? Curr Opin Pharmacol 2008;8:677–84.

43. DeVault KR, Talley NJ. Insights into the future of gastric acid suppression. Nat Rev Gastroenterol Hepatol 2009;6:524–32.

44. Howden CW, Ballard ED, Koch FK, et al. Control of 24-hour intragastric acidity with morning dosing of immediate-release and delayed-release proton pump inhibitors in patients with GERD. J Clin Gastroenterol 2009;43:323–6.

45. Katz PO. Review article: putting immediate-release proton-pump inhibitors into clinical practice–improving nocturnal acid control and avoiding the possible complications of excessive acid exposure. Aliment Pharmacol Ther 2005;22(Suppl 3): 31–8.

46. Howden CW. Review article: immediate-release proton-pump inhibitor therapy–potential advantages. Aliment Pharmacol Ther 2005;22(Suppl 3): 25–30.

47. Katz PO, Koch FK, Ballard ED, et al. Comparison of the effects of immediate-release omeprazole oral suspension, delayed-release lansoprazole capsules and delayed-release esomeprazole capsules on nocturnal gastric acidity after bedtime dosing in patients with night-time GERD symptoms. Aliment Pharmacol Ther 2007;25:197–205.

48. Gralnek IM, Dulai GS, Fennerty MB, et al. Esomeprazole versus other proton pump inhibitors in erosive esophagitis: a meta-analysis of randomized clinical trials. Clin Gastroenterol Hepatol 2006;4:1452–8.

49. Kahrilas PJ, Falk GW, Johnson DA, et al. Esomeprazole improves healing and symptom resolution as compared with omeprazole in reflux oesophagitis patients: a randomized controlled trial—the esomeprazole study investigators. Aliment Pharmacol Ther 2000;14:1249–58.

50. Richter JE, Kahrilas PJ, Johanson J, et al. Efficacy and safety of esomeprazole compared with omeprazole in GERD patients with erosive esophagitis: a randomized controlled trial. Am J Gastroenterol 2001;96:656–65.

51. Castell DO, Kahrilas PJ, Richter JE, et al. Esomeprazole (40 mg) compared with lansoprazole (30 mg) in the treatment of erosive esophagitis. Am J Gastroenterol 2002;97:575–83.

52. Labenz J, Armstrong D, Lauritsen K, et al. A randomized comparative study of esomeprazole 40 mg versus pantoprazole 40 mg for healing erosive oesophagitis: the EXPO study. Aliment Pharmacol Ther 2005;21:739–46.

53. Fennerty MB, Johanson JF, Hwang C, et al. Efficacy of esomeprazole 40 mg vs. lansoprazole 30 mg for healing moderate to severe erosive oesophagitis. Aliment Pharmacol Ther 2005;21:455–63.

54. Sharma P, Shaheen NJ, Perez MC, et al. Healing of erosive oesophagitis with dexlansoprazole MR, a proton pump inhibitor with a novel dual delayed release formulation: results from two randomized controlled studies. Aliment Pharmacol Ther 2009; 29:731–41.

55. Metz DC, Howden CW, Pere MC, et al. Clinical trial: dexlansoprazole MR, a proton pump inhibitor with dual delayed-release technology, effectively controls symptoms and prevents relapse in patients with healed erosive oesophagitis. Aliment Pharmacol Ther 2009;29:742–54.

56. Fass R, Chey WD, Zakko SF, et al. Clinical trial: the effects of the proton pump inhibitor dexlansoprazole MR on daytime and nighttime heartburn in patients with non-erosive reflux disease. Aliment Pharmacol Ther 2009;29:1261–72.

57. Howden CW, Larsen LM, Perez MC, et al. Clinical trial: efficacy and safety of dexlansoprazole MR 60 and 90 mg in healed erosive oesophagitis–maintenance of healing and symptom relief. Aliment Pharmacol Ther 2009;30:895–907.

58. Pai VG, Pai NV, Thacker HP, et al. Comparative clinical trial of S-pantoprazole versus racemic pantoprazole in the treatment of gastro-esophageal reflux disease. World J Gastroenterol 2006;12: 6017–20.

59. Pai V, Pai N. A randomized, double-blind, comparative study of dexrabeprazole 10 mg versus rabeprazole 20 mg in the treatment of gastroesophageal reflux disease. World J Gastroenterol 2007;13:4100–2.

60. Zhou Q, Yan XF, Pan WS, et al. Is the required therapeutic effect always achieved by racemic switch of proton-pump inhibitors? World J Gastroenterol 2008;14:2617–9.

61. Periclou AP, Goldwater R, Lee SM, et al. A comparative pharmacodynamic study of IY-81149 versus omeprazole in patients with gastroesophageal reflux disease. Clin Pharmacol Ther 2000;68:304–11.

62. Galmiche JP, Bruley Des Varannes S, Ducrotte P, et al. Tenatoprazole, a novel proton pump inhibitor with a prolonged plasma half-life: effects on intragastric pH and comparison with esomeprazole in healthy volunteers. Aliment Pharmacol Ther 2004; 19:655–62.

63. Galmiche JP, Sacher-Huvelin S, Bruley des Varannes S, et al. A comparative study of the early effects of tenatoprazole 40 mg and esomeprazole 40 mg on intragastric pH in healthy volunteers. Aliment Pharmacol Ther 2005;21:575–82.

64. Hunt RH, Armstrong D, James C, et al. Effect on intragastric pH of a PPI with a prolonged plasma half-life: comparison between tenatoprazole and esomeprazole on the duration of acid suppression in healthy male volunteers. Am J Gastroenterol 2005;100:1949–56.

65. Thomson AB, Cohen P, Ficheux H, et al. Comparison of the effects of fasting morning, fasting evening and fed bedtime administration of tenatoprazole on intragastric pH in healthy volunteers: a randomized three-way crossover study. Aliment Pharmacol Ther 2006;23:1179–87.

66. Hunt RH, Armstrong D, Yaghoobi M, et al. Pharmacodynamics and pharmacokinetics of S-tenatoprazole-Na 30 mg, 60 mg and 90 mg versus esomeprazole 40 mg in healthy male subjects. Aliment Pharmacol Ther 2010;31:648–57.

67. Yuan Y, Chen Y, Hunt RH. Dose-effect of S-tenatoprazole-Na in healthy volunteers: a meta-analysis of individual subject data from four pharmacodynamic studies [abstract: S1093]. Gastroenterology 2008;134(Suppl 1):A176.

68. Asano S, Yoshida A, Yashiro H, et al. The cavity structure for docking the K(+)-competitive inhibitors in the gastric proton pump. J Biol Chem 2004;279:13968–75.

69. Nilsson C, Albrektson E, Rydholm H, et al. Tolerability, pharmacokinetics and effects on gastric acid secretion after single oral doses of the potassium-competitive acid blocker AZD0865 in healthy male subjects [abstract]. Gastroenterology 2009;128(4 Suppl 2):A528.

70. Yu KS, Bae KS, Shon JH, et al. Pharmacokinetic and pharmacodynamic evaluation of a novel proton pump inhibitor, YH1885, in healthy volunteers. J Clin Pharmacol 2004;44:73–82.

71. Gedda K, Briving C, Svensson K, et al. Mechanism of action of AZD0865, a K+-competitive inhibitor of gastric H+, K+-ATPase. Biochem Pharmacol 2007; 73:198–205.

72. Ito K, Kinoshita K, Tomizawa A, et al. Pharmacological profile of novel acid pump antagonist 7-(4-fluorobenzyloxy)-2,3-dimethyl-1-{[(1S,2S)-2-methyl cyclopropyl]methyl}-1H-pyrrolo [2,3-d]pyridazine (CS-526). J Pharmacol Exp Ther 2007;323:308–17.

73. Ito K, Kinoshita K, Tomizawa A, et al. The effect of subchronic administration of 7-(4-fluorobenzyloxy)-2,3-dimethyl-1-{[(1S,2S)-2 methylcyclopropyl] methyl}-1H-pyrrolo[2,3-d]pyridazine (CS-526), a novel acid pump antagonist, on gastric acid secretion and gastrin levels in rats. J Pharmacol Exp Ther 2008; 326:163–70.

74. Simon WA, Herrmann M, Klein T, et al. Soraprazan: setting new standards in inhibition of gastric acid secretion. J Pharmacol Exp Ther 2007;321:866–74.

75. Kahrilas PJ, Dent J, Lauritsen K, et al. A randomized, comparative trial of three doses of AZD0865 and esomeprazole for healing of reflux esophagitis. Clin Gastroenterol Hepatol 2007;5: 1385–91.

76. Dent J, Kahrilas PJ, Hatlebakk J, et al. A randomized, comparative trial of a potassium-competitive acid blocker (AZD0865) and esomeprazole for the treatment of patients with nonerosive reflux disease. Am J Gastroenterol 2008;103:20–6.

77. Tran T, Lowry AM, El-Serag HB. Meta-analysis: the efficacy of over-the-counter gastroesophageal reflux disease therapies. Aliment Pharmacol Ther 2007;25:143–53.

78. Armstrong D, Marshall JK, Chiba N, et al. Canadian Consensus Conference on the management of gastroesophageal reflux disease in adults– Update 2004. Can J Gastroenterol 2005;19:15–35.

79. Scarpignato C, Galmiche JP. The role of H2-receptor antagonists in the era of proton pump inhibitors. In: Lundell L, editor. Guidelines for management of symptomatic gastro-oesophageal reflux disease. London: Science Press; 1998. p. 55–66.

80. Rackoff A, Agrawal A, Hila A, et al. Histamine-2 receptor antagonists at night improve gastroesophageal reflux disease symptoms for patients on proton pump inhibitor therapy. Dis Esophagus 2005;18:370–3.

81. Xue S, Katz PO, Banerjee P, et al. Bedtime H2 blockers improve nocturnal gastric acid control in GERD patients on proton pump inhibitors. Aliment Pharmacol Ther 2001;15:1351–6.

82. Ours T, Fackler W, Richter J, et al. Nocturnal acid breakthrough: clinical significance and correlation with esophageal acid exposure. Am J Gastroenterol 2003;98:545–50.

83. Fandriks L, Lonroth H, Pettersson A, et al. Can famotidine and omeprazole be combined on a once-daily basis? Scand J Gastroenterol 2007;42:689–94.

84. Ang D, Blondeau K, Sifrim D, et al. The spectrum of motor function abnormalities in gastroesophageal reflux disease and Barrett's esophagus. Digestion 2009;79:158–68.

85. Fass R, Sifrim D. Management of heartburn not responding to proton pump inhibitors. Gut 2009;58: 295–309.

86. Champion G, Richter JE, Singh S, et al. Effects of oral erythromycin on esophageal pH and pressure profiles in patients with gastroesophageal reflux disease. Dig Dis Sci 1994;39:129–37.

87. Chaussade S, Michopoulos S, Sogni P, et al. Motilin agonist erythromycin increases human lower esophageal sphincter pressure by stimulation of cholinergic nerves. Dig Dis Sci 1994;39:381–4.

88. Chrysos E, Tzovaras G, Epanomeritakis E, et al. Erythromycin enhances oesophageal motility in patients with gastro-oesophageal reflux. ANZ J Surg 2001;71:98–102.

89. Finizia C, Lundell L, Cange L, et al. The effect of cisapride on oesophageal motility and lower sphincter function in patients with gastro-oesophageal reflux disease. Eur J Gastroenterol Hepatol 2002;14:9–14.

90. Fox M, Menne D, Stutz B, et al. The effects of tegaserod on oesophageal function and bolus transport

in healthy volunteers: studies using concurrent high-resolution manometry and videofluoroscopy. Aliment Pharmacol Ther 2006;24:1017–27.

91. Greenwood B, Dieckman D, Kirst HA, et al. Effects of LY267108, an erythromycin analogue derivative, on lower esophageal sphincter function in the cat. Gastroenterology 1994;106:624–8.

92. Inauen W, Emde C, Weber B, et al. Effects of ranitidine and cisapride on acid reflux and oesophageal motility in patients with reflux oesophagitis: a 24 hour ambulatory combined pH and manometry study. Gut 1993;34:1025–31.

93. Kahrilas PJ, Quigley EM, Castell DO, et al. The effects of tegaserod (HTF 919) on oesophageal acid exposure in gastro-oesophageal reflux disease. Aliment Pharmacol Ther 2000;14:1503–9.

94. Mertens V, Blondeau K, Pauwels A, et al. Azithromycin reduces gastroesophageal reflux and aspiration in lung transplant recipients. Dig Dis Sci 2009;54:972–9.

95. Peeters TL. Erythromycin and other macrolides as prokinetic agents. Gastroenterology 1993;105:1886–99.

96. Staiano A, Clouse RE. The effects of cisapride on the topography of oesophageal peristalsis. Aliment Pharmacol Ther 1996;10:875–82.

97. Tack J. Prokinetics and fundic relaxants in upper functional GI disorders. Curr Opin Pharmacol 2008;8:690–6.

98. Gardner JD, Rodriguez-Stanley S, Robinson M, et al. Cisapride inhibits meal-stimulated gastric acid secretion and post-prandial gastric acidity in subjects with gastro-oesophageal reflux disease. Aliment Pharmacol Ther 2002;16:1819–29.

99. Abdulnour-Nakhoul S, Tobey NA, Nakhoul NL, et al. The effect of tegaserod on esophageal submucosal glands bicarbonate and mucin secretion. Dig Dis Sci 2008;53:2366–72.

100. Majewski M, Jaworski T, Sarosiek I, et al. Significant enhancement of esophageal pre-epithelial defense by tegaserod: implications for an esophagoprotective effect. Clin Gastroenterol Hepatol 2007;5:430–8.

101. Peeters TL. Old and new targets for prokinetic drugs: motilin and ghrelin receptors. Eur Rev Med Pharmacol Sci 2008;12(Suppl 1):136–7.

102. Sanger GJ. Motilin, ghrelin and related neuropeptides as targets for the treatment of GI diseases. Drug Discov Today 2008;13:234–9.

103. Tomita R, Tanjoh K, Munakata K. The role of motilin and cisapride in the enteric nervous system of the lower esophageal sphincter in humans. Surg Today 1997;27:985–92.

104. Netzer P, Schmitt B, Inauen W. Effects of ABT-229, a motilin agonist, on acid reflux, oesophageal motility and gastric emptying in patients with gastro-oesophageal reflux disease. Aliment Pharmacol Ther 2002;16:1481–90.

105. van Herwaarden MA, Samsom M, Van Nispen CH, et al. The effect of motilin agonist ABT-229 on gastro-oesophageal reflux, oesophageal motility and lower oesophageal sphincter characteristics in GERD patients. Aliment Pharmacol Ther 2000;14:453–62.

106. Pennathur A, Tran A, Cioppi M, et al. Erythromycin strengthens the defective lower esophageal sphincter in patients with gastroesophageal reflux disease. Am J Surg 1994;167:169–72.

107. Mitselos A, Peeters TL, Depoortere I. Desensitization and internalization of the human motilin receptor is independent of the C-terminal tail. Peptides 2008;29:1167–75.

108. Dodds WJ, Dent J, Hogan WJ, et al. Mechanisms of gastroesophageal reflux in patients with reflux esophagitis. N Engl J Med 1982;307:1547–52.

109. Holloway RH, Penagini R, Ireland AC. Criteria for objective definition of transient lower esophageal sphincter relaxation. Am J Physiol 1995;268:G128–33.

110. Hirsch DP, Tytgat GN, Boeckxstaens GE. Transient lower oesophageal sphincter relaxations–a pharmacological target for gastro-oesophageal reflux disease? Aliment Pharmacol Ther 2002;16:17–26.

111. Janssens J, Sifrim D. Spontaneous transient lower esophageal sphincter relaxations: a target for treatment of gastroesophageal reflux disease. Gastroenterology 1995;109:1703–6.

112. Mittal RK, McCallum RW. Characteristics of transient lower esophageal sphincter relaxation in humans. Am J Physiol 1987;252:G636–41.

113. Sifrim D, Holloway R. Transient lower esophageal sphincter relaxations: how many or how harmful? Am J Gastroenterol 2001;96:2529–32.

114. Beaumont H, Bennink RJ, de JJ, et al. The position of the acid pocket as a major risk factor for acidic reflux in healthy subjects and patients with GORD. Gut 2010;59:441–51.

115. Cange L, Johnsson E, Rydholm H, et al. Baclofen-mediated gastro-oesophageal acid reflux control in patients with established reflux disease. Aliment Pharmacol Ther 2002;16:869–73.

116. Ciccaglione AF, Marzio L. Effect of acute and chronic administration of the GABA B agonist baclofen on 24 hour pH metry and symptoms in control subjects and in patients with gastro-oesophageal reflux disease. Gut 2003;52:464–70.

117. Koek GH, Sifrim D, Lerut T, et al. Effect of the GABA(B) agonist baclofen in patients with symptoms and duodeno-gastro-oesophageal reflux refractory to proton pump inhibitors. Gut 2003;52:1397–402.

118. Lidums I, Lehmann A, Checklin H, et al. Control of transient lower esophageal sphincter relaxations and reflux by the GABA(B) agonist baclofen in normal subjects. Gastroenterology 2000;118:7–13.

119. van Herwaarden MA, Samsom M, Rydholm H, et al. The effect of baclofen on gastro-oesophageal

reflux, lower oesophageal sphincter function and reflux symptoms in patients with reflux disease. Aliment Pharmacol Ther 2002;16:1655–62.

120. Vela MF, Tutuian R, Katz PO, et al. Baclofen decreases acid and non-acid post-prandial gastro-oesophageal reflux measured by combined multichannel intraluminal impedance and pH. Aliment Pharmacol Ther 2003;17:243–51.

121. Zhang Q, Lehmann A, Rigda R, et al. Control of transient lower oesophageal sphincter relaxations and reflux by the GABA(B) agonist baclofen in patients with gastro-oesophageal reflux disease. Gut 2002;50:19–24.

122. Boeckxstaens GE, Rydholm H, Lei A, et al. Effect of lesogaberan, a novel GABA-receptor agonist, on transient lower esophageal sphincter relaxations in male subjects. Aliment Pharmacol Ther 2010; 31:1208–17.

123. Omari TI, Benninga MA, Sansom L, et al. Effect of baclofen on esophagogastric motility and gastro-esophageal reflux in children with gastroesophageal reflux disease: a randomized controlled trial. J Pediatr 2006;149:468–74.

124. Beaumont H, Jonsson-Rylander AC, Carlsson K, et al. The role of GABA(A) receptors in the control of transient lower oesophageal sphincter relaxations in the dog. Br J Pharmacol 2008;153: 1195–202.

125. Boeckxstaens GE, Hirsch DP, Fakhry N, et al. Involvement of cholecystokininA receptors in transient lower esophageal sphincter relaxations triggered by gastric distension. Am J Gastroenterol 1998;93:1823–8.

126. Penagini R, Bianchi PA. Effect of morphine on gastroesophageal reflux and transient lower esophageal sphincter relaxation. Gastroenterology 1997;113:409–14.

127. Hirsch DP, Tytgat GN, Boeckxstaens GE. Is glutamate involved in transient lower esophageal sphincter relaxations? Dig Dis Sci 2002;47:661–6.

128. Lehmann A, Blackshaw LA, Branden L, et al. Cannabinoid receptor agonism inhibits transient lower esophageal sphincter relaxations and reflux in dogs. Gastroenterology 2002;123:1129–34.

129. Beaumont H, Jensen J, Carlsson A, et al. Effect of delta9-tetrahydrocannabinol, a cannabinoid receptor agonist, on the triggering of transient lower oesophageal sphincter relaxations in dogs and humans. Br J Pharmacol 2009;156:153–62.

130. Frisby CL, Mattsson JP, Jensen JM, et al. Inhibition of transient lower esophageal sphincter relaxation and gastroesophageal reflux by metabotropic glutamate receptor ligands. Gastroenterology 2005;129:995–1004.

131. Keywood C, Wakefield M, Tack J. A proof-of-concept study evaluating the effect of ADX10059, a metabotropic glutamate receptor-5 negative allosteric modulator, on acid exposure and symptoms in gastro-oesophageal reflux disease. Gut 2009;58:1192–9.

132. Hirsch DP, Holloway RH, Tytgat GN, et al. Involvement of nitric oxide in human transient lower esophageal sphincter relaxations and esophageal primary peristalsis. Gastroenterology 1998;115: 1374–80.

133. Lehmann A, Antonsson M, Bremner-Danielsen M, et al. Activation of the GABA(B) receptor inhibits transient lower esophageal sphincter relaxations in dogs. Gastroenterology 1999;117:1147–54.

134. Grossi L, Spezzaferro M, Sacco LF, et al. Effect of baclofen on oesophageal motility and transient lower oesophageal sphincter relaxations in GORD patients: a 48-h manometric study. Neurogastroenterol Motil 2008;20:760–6.

135. Beaumont H, Boeckxstaens GE. Does the presence of a hiatal hernia affect the efficacy of the reflux inhibitor baclofen during add-on therapy? Am J Gastroenterol 2009;104:1764–71.

136. Gerson LB, Huff FJ, Hila A, et al. Arbaclofen placarbil decreases postprandial reflux in patients with gastroesophageal reflux disease. Am J Gastroenterol 2010;105:1266–75.

137. Lehmann A, Brändén L, Carlsson A, et al. AZD3355, a novel GABAB receptor agonist inhibits transient lower esophageal sphincter relaxation in the dog (Abstract). Gastroenterology 2008;134: A49–50.

138. Boeckxstaens GE, Beaumont H, Hatlebakk JG, et al. Efficacy and tolerability of the novel reflux inhibitor, AZD3355, as add-on treatment in GERD patients with symptoms despite proton pump inhibitor therapy [abstract]. Gastroenterology 2009;136:A436.

139. Jensen J, Lehmann A, Uvebrant A, et al. Transient lower esophageal sphincter relaxations in dogs are inhibited by a metabotropic glutamate receptor 5 antagonist. Eur J Pharmacol 2005;519: 154–7.

140. Zerbib F, Keywood C, Strabach G. Efficacy, tolerability and pharmacokinetics of a modified release formulation of ADX10059, a negative allosteric modulator of metabotropic glutamate receptor 5: an esophageal pH-impedance study in healthy subjects. Neurogastroenterol Motil 2010;22(8): 859–65, e231.

141. Partosoedarso ER, Abrahams TP, Scullion RT, et al. Cannabinoid1 receptor in the dorsal vagal complex modulates lower oesophageal sphincter relaxation in ferrets. J Physiol 2003;550:149–58.

142. Vela MF, Camacho-Lobato L, Srinivasan R, et al. Simultaneous intraesophageal impedance and pH measurement of acid and nonacid gastroesophageal reflux: effect of omeprazole. Gastroenterology 2001;120:1599–606.

143. Clouse RE, Lustman PJ, Eckert TC, et al. Low-dose trazodone for symptomatic patients with esophageal contraction abnormalities. A double-blind, placebo-controlled trial. Gastroenterology 1987; 92:1027–36.

144. Handa M, Mine K, Yamamoto H, et al. Antidepressant treatment of patients with diffuse esophageal spasm: a psychosomatic approach. J Clin Gastroenterol 1999;28:228–32.

145. Tack J, Sarnelli G. Serotonergic modulation of visceral sensation: upper gastrointestinal tract. Gut 2002;51(Suppl 1):i77–80.

146. Sarkar S, Aziz Q, Woolf CJ, et al. Contribution of central sensitisation to the development of noncardiac chest pain. Lancet 2000;356:1154–9.

147. Sarkar S, Hobson AR, Hughes A, et al. The prostaglandin E2 receptor-1 (EP-1) mediates acid-induced visceral pain hypersensitivity in humans. Gastroenterology 2003;124:18–25.

148. Willert RP, Woolf CJ, Hobson AR, et al. The development and maintenance of human visceral pain hypersensitivity is dependent on the N-methyl-D-aspartate receptor. Gastroenterology 2004;126:683–92.

149. Orlando RC, Turjman NA, Tobey NA, et al. Mucosal protection by sucralfate and its components in acid-exposed rabbit esophagus. Gastroenterology 1987;93:352–61.

150. Farré R, Cardozo L, Blondeau K, et al. Esophageal mucosal damage induced by weakly acidic solutions containing unconjugated bile acids, similar to reflux in GERD patients "on" PPI, can be prevented with anti-oxidants [abstract]. Gastroenterology 2009;136:A16.

151. Lauritsen K, Deviere J, Bigard MA, et al. Esomeprazole 20 mg and lansoprazole 15 mg in maintaining healed reflux oesophagitis: metropole study results. Aliment Pharmacol Ther 2003;17:333–41.

152. Labenz J, Armstrong D, Lauritsen K, et al. Esomeprazole 20 mg vs. pantoprazole 20 mg for maintenance therapy of healed erosive oesophagitis: results from the EXPO study. Aliment Pharmacol Ther 2005;22:803–11.

153. Boeckxstaens GE. Reflux inhibitors: a new approach for GERD? Curr Opin Pharmacol 2008;8:1–5.

154. Johnson DA, Levy BH III. Evolving drugs in gastroesophageal reflux disease: pharmacological treatment beyond proton pump inhibitors. Expert Opin Pharmacother 2010;11:1541–8.

155. Bytzer P, Christensen PB, Damkier P, et al. Adenocarcinoma of the esophagus and Barrett's esophagus: a population-based study. Am J Gastroenterol 1999;94:86–91.

156. Jones R, Armstrong D, Malfertheiner P, et al. Does the treatment of gastroesophageal reflux disease (GERD) meet patients' needs? A survey-based study. Curr Med Res Opin 2006;22:657–62.

157. Armstrong D. Symptom assessment – methods and content. J Clin Gastroenterol 2007;41(S2):S184–92.

158. Armstrong D. A critical assessment of the current state of NERD. Digestion 2008;1(Suppl 1):46–54.

159. Poh C, Gasiorowska A, Fass R, et al. Upper GI tract findings in patients with heartburn in whom proton pump inhibitor treatment failed versus those not receiving antireflux treatment. Gastrointest Endosc 2010;71:28–34.

160. Miner P, Katz O, Chen Y, et al. Gastric acid control with esomeprazole, lansoprazole, omeprazole, pantoprazole and rabeprazole: a five-way crossover study. Am J Gastroenterol 2003;98:2616–20.

161. Khuroo MS, Yattoo GN, Javid G, et al. A comparison of omeprazole and placebo for bleeding peptic ulcer. N Engl J Med 1997;336:1054–8.

162. Metz DC, Soffer E, Forsmark CE, et al. Maintenance oral pantoprazole therapy is effective for patients with Zollinger-Ellison syndrome and idiopathic hypersecretion. Am J Gastroenterol 2003;98:301–7.

163. Bardhan KD, Stanghellini V, Armstrong D, et al. Evaluation of GERD symptoms during therapy Part 1: development of the new GERD questionnaire ReQuest. Digestion 2004;69:229–37.

164. Mönnikes H, Bardhan KD, Stanghellini V, et al. Evaluation of GERD symptoms during therapy Part II: psychometric evaluation and validation of the new questionnaire ReQuest in erosive GERD. Digestion 2004;69:238–44.

The Natural History and Complications of Eosinophilic Esophagitis

Alex Straumann, MD

KEYWORDS

- Esophagitis • Esophageal stricture • GERD • Endoscopy
- Boerhaave's syndrome

Eosinophilic esophagitis (EE) is a relatively newly recognized disorder, with the first comprehensive descriptions of this inflammatory esophageal disease published less than 15 years ago.[1–3] Within this relatively short time frame, EE has become a well-recognized and clearly defined clinicopathologic entity. Symptoms revolve around the esophagus, where eosinophilic accumulation occurs. Long-term administration of proton-pump inhibitors alleviates neither symptoms nor eosinophilia.[4] Initially thought to be a rare curiosity, EE has emerged as one of the most common causes of dysphagia and esophageal food impaction in adults.[5] In children, the latest incidence rates may even exceed those of pediatric inflammatory bowel disease.[6] Despite enormous research activity, the natural history, the long-term prognosis, and the complications of EE still remain poorly understood.[7]

GENERAL CONSIDERATIONS ABOUT THE NATURAL HISTORY OF A DISEASE
Characterization of the Natural History of a Disease

The two terms "natural history" and "natural course" of a disease are used widely in medical literature, but a precise definition is hard to find. A simple paraphrase, "the course of a disease left untreated," is usually accepted as the definition of a disease's natural history. The circumscription, "The natural history of a disease describes the expected course followed by the given disease over time, its characteristic pattern, and its time-intensity gradient," depicts the disease-specific behavior more precisely.

Importance of Knowing the Natural History of a Disease

A PubMed literature search with the key word "natural history" (not specifically of EE) revealed that in 1 single year, 2006, 1651 articles were published on this topic. There are at least three reasons for this proliferation of publications:

1. Research purposes: In the development of any novel medical or surgical strategy, the natural history of the disorder is the benchmark against which the efficacy and safety of all new therapeutic measures are compared.
2. Patient care purposes: Newly confronted with a disease, patients and family members are eager to learn precise information about the disease and its prognosis. Specifically, survival, risk of disability, inability to work, and the impact of the disease on quality of life are topics anxiously explored in the search for information about the disease's natural history. For treating physicians, knowing the particular disease behavior establishes the cornerstone on which counseling and patient care is based.
3. Socioeconomic purposes: For health care institutions, epidemiology services, social institutions, and health and life insurances, knowledge

This article originally appeared in *Gastrointestinal Endoscopy Clinics of North America, volume 18, 2008.*
Department of Gastroenterology, University Hospital Basel, Roemerstrasse 7, 4600 Olten, Switzerland
E-mail address: alex.straumann@hin.ch

Thorac Surg Clin 21 (2011) 575–587
doi:10.1016/j.thorsurg.2011.09.004

of the natural course of a disease is crucial in planning appropriate measures and in estimating the burden of disease, including direct and indirect costs.

Particularities of Natural History Studies

The primary objective of a natural history study is to monitor, as punctiliously as possible, the unaltered course of a specific disease. One could even consider such a study as a clinical trial that has the particularity that no drug is under investigation. Nevertheless, this small difference from therapeutic clinical trials presents relevant practical consequences for executing and evaluating natural history studies.

The main difference between natural history studies and therapeutic clinical trials is the risk for the study participants. Whereas in a therapeutic trial the side effects of the study medication are the main safety concern, in a natural history study a "wait and watch" attitude poses the main risk for participants. If the natural course of a disorder is associated with relevant disturbances, or if the disease has a risk for complications or even for a fatal outcome, ethical considerations prohibit performing such observational studies if an approved treatment is available. Further differences between these two types of study are that the planning and execution of natural history studies are not as rigidly defined or supervised by regulatory authorities as therapeutic trials; fundraising may be difficult because of the lack of commercial interests; and, methodologically, the established study designs have different rankings for their level of evidence.[8]

Designs for Natural History Studies

In general, natural history studies can be performed with study designs that are identical to those for therapeutic clinical trials. In natural history studies, however, the levels of evidence in well-established study designs are different from those seen in clinical trials. The ideal natural history study assesses, in a prospective and controlled fashion, all relevant disease-specific aspects, including survival, factors interfering with the quality of life (eg, pain, dysphagia, diarrhea), general and disease-specific complications, hospitalizations, surgical procedures, absenteeism, and direct and indirect costs. The study should have a disease-adjusted time frame and should include an appropriate number of affected individuals as well as a representative, nonaffected control population. Following increasing levels of evidence, each study design discussed here can be used to assess the natural history of a given disease.[8]

Case reports
Especially for novel diseases, case reports—single-spot observations—may be of importance in drawing attention to a previously unrecognized aspect of a particular disease. Their level of evidence, however, is limited by the risk that the case actually may report a phenomenon not related to, or not even representative of, the particular disease. This study type thus has the lowest level of evidence. Conclusions fashioned from case reports always require confirmation by more robust ascertainments.

Case series
The pooling of observations in case series allows a more precise description of a phenomenon than that provided by a single case report. The weakness of case series is that the documentation of the cases does not follow a previously defined protocol and thus may differ among the study participants. Additionally, case series have an inherent risk of a selection bias with consecutive misinterpretations.

Database analyses
In general, in a database, the information is collected continuously without a predefined goal. Databases therefore contain large amounts of data but pose a difficulty in performing an analysis that focuses on a particular issue. Nevertheless, databases are good instruments for recruiting participants for cohort studies.

Placebo-group analyses
Placebo-controlled trials are well established for assessing the efficacy and safety of new medications. The placebo groups from randomized, double-blind trials are well-defined groups of patients who are followed in accordance with pre-defined protocols. The analysis of a placebo group therefore provides a comprehensive description of the natural history of a given disorder. A placebo-group analysis is the only type of interventional study that can be used to assess the natural history of a disease; all other methods are observational studies. The value of the evidence from this type of study for natural history investigations is not as high as for therapeutic trials, however, because in a particular trial the application of a placebo and the follow-up examinations are interventions that themselves may interfere with the natural course of a disease. Furthermore, clinical trials normally cover only a limited follow-up period, and this period may not be long enough

to assess the course of chronic, long-standing diseases.

Cohort studies

Observational cohort studies are considered the reference standard for natural history studies. In a cohort study, a group of individuals is followed over time, following a previously defined protocol. If therapeutic interventions cannot be avoided during the follow-up period, all medications, hospitalizations, and endoscopic and surgical procedures are recorded. In a classic cohort study, the participants are included in the cohort before the end point of interest (eg, the appearance of EE) occurs. The natural history cohort is an exception to this rule, because all individuals included in the cohort are affected with the given disease. This difference creates the limitation that the description of the natural course lacks a comparison. To eliminate this drawback, a control population of healthy individuals is included, according to a case-control technique. This controlled-cohort type of study has the highest level of evidence among natural history studies. Because these studies are time-consuming, expensive, and limited by ethical considerations, only few natural history studies follow this design.

NATURAL HISTORY OF EOSINOPHILIC ESOPHAGITIS

Which Data Characterize the Natural History of Eosinophilic Esophagitis?

In reading this article, it is important to keep in mind that, to date, only one prospective study describing the natural history of EE has been published.[9] Except for one analysis of a placebo group from the only randomized, double-blind, placebo-controlled therapeutic trial in children,[10] all data cited in this article have been gathered from analyses of case series and case reports. To supplement this limited information and to illustrate specific points, the author has included a few unpublished observations from the EE clinic at the Kantonsspital Olten, which has provided care for more than 200 adult patients who had EE referred from throughout Switzerland.

Which Parameters Reflect the Activity of Eosinophilic Esophagitis?

Clinicopathologically, EE is characterized by esophageal symptoms and a dense esophageal eosinophilia, both of which persist despite prolonged treatment with proton-pump inhibitors or in the face of normal pH monitoring of the distal esophagus.[4,11] Of note, EE cannot be defined using endoscopic findings: the diagnostic value of endoscopy is limited because eosinophilic inflammation evokes a variety of mucosal abnormalities, not a single cardinal sign or characteristic pattern.[12,13] (See the article by Fox elsewhere in this issue.)

The clinical part of the EE definition is reflected by esophageal symptoms that vary according to the age of the patient. In adolescents and adults, dysphagia for solid food, starting as an unpleasant feeling during swallowing and escalating to food impaction, is the leading manifestation of EE.[1–3,14] In addition, a considerable subset of patients suffers from retrosternal pain that is independent of the swallowing act. This pain sometimes is induced by imbibing alcoholic beverages, white wine in particular. Pediatric patients who have EE show a broader spectrum of symptoms, including vomiting, abdominal pain, chest pain, dysphagia, food impaction, failure to thrive, and symptoms mimicking gastroesophageal reflux disease (GERD).[4,15] (See the article by Putnam elsewhere in this issue.)

The previously published (and subsequently slightly modified) grading score (**Box 1**) has proven to be a useful instrument in assessing the severity of the clinical aspects of EE in both practice and research.[9] Because patients who have EE naturally adapt their eating habits to avoid difficulty in swallowing, they must be instructed to answer the questions as if they exercised completely "normal" eating habits, without any restrictions or precautions. The severity of the dysphagia attacks also may vary within any individual patient. Patients thus should be instructed to list their "typical" attack, one which corresponds to their most common and frequently occurring attack. This grading score is of limited value in pediatric settings, because children present a wider spectrum of EE symptoms[15,16] and cannot express their discomfort as discernibly as adolescents or adults. (See the article by Putnam elsewhere in this issue.)

The pathology part of the EE characterization is reflected by distinct histopathologic alterations. (See the article by Collins elsewhere in this issue.)

WHAT IS KNOWN ABOUT THE NATURAL HISTORY OF EOSINOPHILIC ESOPHAGITIS?

Eosinophilic Esophagitis is a Chronic Disease

Even the initial comprehensive descriptions of EE intimated the chronicity of this disorder; indeed, patients often recounted a history of dysphagia that had lasted for years before the diagnosis of EE was finally established.[1,3] As illustration, in the author and colleagues' first case series from 1994, patients had suffered from swallowing

---

Box 1
Grading score for symptoms of eosinophilic esophagitis in adults

Frequency of dysphagia events

No dysphagia events

Once per month

Once per week

Several times per week

Once per day

Several times daily

Duration of dysphagia events

None

Less than 10 seconds

More than 10 seconds to 1 minute

More than 1 to 10 minutes

More than 10 to 60 minutes

More than 60 minutes

Intensity of dysphagia events

Swallowing unhindered without pain

Spontaneous passage with a slight feeling of retrosternal resistance (food passage without delay)

Spontaneous passage with a feeling of retching (food passage with a short delay)

Forced anterograde passage (short periods of obstruction, necessitating intervention, such as drinking)

Forced retrograde removal (complete obstruction, removable only by vomiting or retching)

Necessity for endoscopic intervention (continuous obstruction, not removable by patient)

Presence of retrosternal pain not related to swallowing (occurring spontaneously or alcohol-induced)

No pain

Once per month

Once per week

Several times per week

Once per day

Several times daily

---

disturbances for an average of 4.3 years (range, 1–13 years) before receiving the diagnosis of EE.[3] A second indicator of the chronic nature of EE was the observation that relapses in symptoms and eosinophilic inflammation frequently occurred after the cessation of therapy. In one therapeutic study from Australia, 14 of 19 patients (74%) experienced a relapse within 3 months after cessation of successful topical corticosteroid treatment.[14] Additional evidence that EE is a chronic disease was furnished by one study that focused primarily on the natural history in which 30 adults were followed for an average of 7 years.[9] The vast majority of the patients had persistent dysphagia over years, with a significant impact on the quality of life. This analysis further demonstrated that the eosinophilic infiltration persisted in all symptomatic patients.

Nevertheless, one important uncertainty remains, and that is whether children who have EE grow up to become adults who have EE or whether this chronic inflammation can be outgrown. Unfortunately the natural history of EE has not been followed in children, but several observations indicate that the pediatric form of EE is clinically and histologically like the adult form, a chronic disease. For instance, it is common for children who have EE to have a parent with a long-standing history of dysphagia or even with documented esophageal strictures. In some cases, examination of esophageal biopsy slides from the parent reveals evidence of long-standing esophageal eosinophilia.[17] In addition, the phenomenon of symptom and inflammation relapse after cessation of successful treatment is as common in children as it is in adults[16] EE thus is currently considered a chronic disorder and harbors, if untreated, the potential and yet unmeasured risks of uncontrolled and persistent inflammatory process.

The Activity of Eosinophilic Esophagitis May Fluctuate Spontaneously

In general, a chronic disease has the potential to follow several courses. (1) It may resolve spontaneously after a certain time with permanent resolution. (2) It may enter a temporary remission with subsequent relapse. (3) It may progress to a fixed stable state (burned out, but still abnormal). (4) It may follow a relentless progression.

Based on clinical observations, patients who have EE have a waxing and waning course that can occur independent of any therapeutic intervention. The analysis of the placebo group from a therapeutic trial investigating the efficacy of fluticasone propionate in pediatric patients who had EE provides evidence of the spontaneously occurring fluctuations in disease activity.[10] Fifteen children who had active EE, defined as having a peak infiltration of 24 or more eosinophils per high-power field (HPF) in the esophageal mucosa, were assigned randomly to receive placebo and served as untreated controls for the fluticasone group. At study end, 11 placebo patients could be analyzed. Among these 11 patients inhaling placebo, 1 (9%) achieved histologic remission, and 3 (27%) experienced resolution of vomiting during the 3-month study period. This trial thus demonstrates that, in children, EE may resolve spontaneously, at least for a limited time. **Fig. 1** demonstrates that fluctuation in the disease activity occurs in adults as well.

The Activity of Eosinophilic Esophagitis May Fluctuate Depending on Exogenous Allergens

In contrast to the established experience that the natural course of EE is independent of exogenous factors, at least one environmental factor may influence the activity of EE. Fogg and coworkers[18] reported a 21-year-old female patient who had EE and concomitant allergic asthma and rhinitis, with a worsening of symptoms during the pollen season. They further documented that the eosinophilic infiltration in the esophageal tissue paralleled the clinical course: symptoms and eosinophils were almost absent during the winter season, but both symptoms and inflammation relapsed during the pollen season. This case, together with a report of seasonal variation in EE incidence, with the lowest diagnostic rate during the winter period when the levels of outdoor allergens are low,[19] indicates that inhalant allergens may play a pathogenic role in the development of EE.

Eosinophilic Esophagitis Does Not Seem to Limit Life Expectancy

When one is confronted with a new disease, the first crucial question usually focuses on life expectancy and, in particular, on the risk of a fatal outcome. In the 11.5-year follow-up study by the author and colleagues,[9] all 30 adults survived in good health and with stable nutrition. Furthermore, in their database of more than 200 adolescents or adult patients during the last 17 years, no EE-related death has been registered. This information concurs with the current literature that reports no fatal outcomes for patients who have EE. Nevertheless, the observation period for EE is still too short to make definitive statements regarding long-term survival.

Eosinophilic Esophagitis Impairs the Quality of Life

Eating and drinking replenish nutrients and also constitute fundamental pleasures in life. Esophageal disorders therefore may impinge substantially on the quality of life. In their study investigating the potential impact that EE exerted on social and professional activities (ie, on the quality of life), the author and colleagues[9] used a structured interview format. In half of the patients, the dysphagia led to minor lifestyle changes, such as influencing menu choices with respect to food texture, consistently avoiding ingestion of solid foods without simultaneously imbibing liquids, or eschewing eating in restaurants. One of the 30 study participants (3%), a traveling engineer with many customer contacts who needed to eat frequently in restaurants, described how the disease exerted such a major impact on his life that he ultimately had to change jobs. For the remaining 14 patients (47%), the dysphagia exerted no impact on lifestyle.

In summary, EE substantially influences the quality of life in many adults, but most patients learn

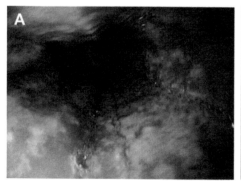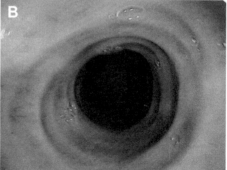

Fig. 1. Spontaneous fluctuation in eosinophilic esophagitis activity. Endoscopic pictures from a 45-year-old man who had a history of dysphagia commencing in 1998 and a diagnosis of EE in 2000. (*A*) An endoscopy performed during a symptomatic relapse revealed a severely inflamed esophageal mucosa covered with white exudates and more than 150 eosinophils per HPF. The patient was screened for a therapeutic trial and received no treatment. The dysphagia then disappeared spontaneously. (*B*) The examination performed 3 months later, during pollen season, revealed that the mucosa had resolution of the acute exudates and the presence of several corrugated rings. Histology revealed a peak infiltration of 12 eosinophils per HPF, a level that did not fulfill the established diagnostic criteria of EE.

to cope with their symptoms. For children, no solid data specifically investigating this subject are available, but it can be speculated that, because of their more severe symptoms, the often imposed dietary restrictions, and the ensuing social consequences, the negative impact on quality of life probably is much greater in children than in adults.[16,20]

Eosinophilic Esophagitis is a Disease Restricted to the Esophagus

To date, almost all reported patients who have EE suffer from an isolated esophageal disease, and esophageal involvement (eg, as is seen with eosinophilic gastroenteritis) tends to be the exception rather than the rule.[2,21,22] It has been shown, however, that in patients who have well-documented EE restricted to the esophagus, peripheral blood eosinophils are able to produce and release functional interleukin-13, and EE must be considered as being, at least in part, a systemic disorder.[23] This consideration prompted the author and colleagues to examine whether a spread from the esophagus-limited EE to eosinophilic gastroenteritis or to an idiopathic hypereosinophilic syndrome could occur and whether EE might be the beginning of a gastrointestinal or even systemic eosinophilic disorder. Endoscopically and histologically, these investigators found no signs of an eosinophilic gastritis or duodenitis. The laboratory tests revealed no abnormalities with respect to hepatic or pancreatic inflammation, and none of the patients developed a persistent, severe eosinophilia in the peripheral blood or an expansion of abnormal T-cell clones. In the ensuing follow-up period, the eosinophilic inflammation has remained limited to the esophagus in all patients.[9] Based on clinical experience and the literature to date, EE is a disease that does not transition to eosinophilic gastroenteritis or other diseases but remains limited to the esophagus. If new symptoms develop, or mucosal eosinophilia is identified in other parts of the gastrointestinal tract, alternative diagnostic possibilities should be reconsidered.

Eosinophilic Esophagitis May Lead to a Remodeling of the Esophagus

From other disorders, such as asthma, it is well known that chronic and persistent eosinophilic inflammation can induce irreversible structural changes in the affected organ.[24] In asthma, this so-called "remodeling" refers to structural changes that include subepithelial fibrosis and angiogenesis, leading finally to a loss of function.[24] Transforming growth factor beta 1 (TGF-β1) plays a crucial role in this process, because patients who have asthma have elevated levels of this profibrotic molecule, and an inhibition of TGF-β1 expression reduces the development of remodeling signs.[25] (See the article by Chehade elsewhere in this issue.)

Murine and translational studies support a role for eosinophils in the development of structural abnormalities observed in the esophageal mucosa.[26] In patients who have EE, the histologic analysis of the subepithelial compartments in the esophagus is hampered because biopsy samples contain almost exclusively epithelial structures. Nonetheless, the author and colleagues obtained adequate subepithelial tissue to permit a representative qualitative analysis in 7 of the 30 patients (23%). In the subepithelial compartments of 6 of these 7 patients (86%), the investigators measured increased fibrous tissue, with thickening and alteration in the subepithelial architecture.[9] This observation has been supported by several later studies that also detected esophageal fibrosis in subepithelial layers.[27–29] For instance, Aceves and colleagues[30] recently identified subepithelial structural alterations in the esophagi of children who had EE. The investigators examined seven children who had a healthy esophagus, seven children who had reflux esophagitis, and seven children who had EE. They found an esophageal mucosa with significantly increased fibrosis, vascularity, and vascular activation in the subepithelial compartment of all patients who had EE. These alterations were not observed in patients who had reflux esophagitis.[30] In contrast to the patients who had GERD and to normal controls, children who had EE demonstrated increased TGF-β1 expression in their esophageal mucosa. It is interesting to speculate that these findings may correspond to endosonographic findings, demonstrating thickened mucosal, submucosal, and muscularis propria layers in the esophagus of patients who have EE.[31]

In summary, the chronic eosinophilic inflammation in EE leads to an irreversible remodeling of the esophagus that probably is responsible for several disease-inherent complications. Whether this process develops in all patients who have EE or whether it occurs in only a subset of patients is not clear, however. It also remains to be determined whether this remodeling is dependent on the activity of the underlying inflammation and whether it can be prevented with therapeutic measures.

Eosinophilic Esophagitis Has Not Been Associated with Increased Risk of Premalignant or Malignant Conditions

Many immune-mediated, chronic, inflammatory diseases of the gastrointestinal tract (eg, chronic-atrophic gastritis and ulcerative colitis) carry an increased risk of developing local malignancies. Furthermore, patients who have chronic eosinophilic disorders are characterized by abnormal T-cell clones and increased risk for lymphoproliferative disorders.[32,33] In the natural history study by the author and colleagues,[9] all patients were examined thoroughly for malignant and premalignant conditions at the site of the inflammation and in the peripheral blood. No malignant tumors or dysplasias were detected in the esophagus, either endoscopically or histologically. Additionally, the flow cytometric analysis of the peripheral lymphocytes did not reveal any evidence of T-cell clones or lymphoproliferative diseases. After 15 years of collective follow-up of 200 patients, no local or systemic premalignant or malignant condition related to EE has been identified, and no case series have been yet reported. The author and colleagues therefore consider the risk for developing malignancies in EE as low, but extended observation is needed before this possibility can be excluded irrefutably.

Predictive Factors for Clinical Course of Patients Who Have Eosinophilic Esophagitis

Two predictive factors have been identified to date. One concerns the natural course, and the other concerns the response to therapy. For adult patients, those who have a peripheral eosinophilia experience more dysphagia attacks during the course of the disease than do those who have normal peripheral blood counts.[9] Children who have IgE-mediated forms of EE do not respond as well to treatment with corticosteroids as do those who have nonallergic forms.[10] It still is too early, however, to define the significance of other potential predictive factors, such as age at presentation, gender, phenotype, or response to treatment.

COMPLICATIONS OF EOSINOPHILIC ESOPHAGITIS

The complications EE can be divided into two categories: complications that are direct sequelae of the uninfluenced (non-intervened) ongoing inflammation and therefore are related to the natural history of EE and complications related to medical or endoscopic interventions.

Disease-Inherent Complications

For many chronic inflammatory disorders (eg, asthma) and noninflammatory disorders (eg, diabetes), the underlying process itself, uninfluenced by intervention, may lead to long-term complications. Because EE is a typical representative of a chronic inflammatory disease, it is not surprising that the inflammation may result in local complications.

Eosinophilic esophagitis may lead to food impaction

Acute food impaction—a primary manifestation of dysphagia—is a leading and common complication of EE in children[15] as well as in adults.[14,27] For example, 17 of 31 adult patients (60%) referred for a diagnostic work-up for food impaction received the diagnosis of EE.[5] This complication may occur at any stage of the disease, as an initial manifestation or after many years of EE duration. The risk of impaction primarily depends on the consistency of the food; particularly problematic are dry rice and fibrous meat (eg, chicken and beef). The first indication is a feeling of retrosternal resistance with a delayed passage of the bolus, precisely at the niveau of the impacted food, immediately followed by hypersalivation. Complete obstruction may resolve spontaneously or persist for hours. If the bolus is impacted in the proximal part of the esophagus, the patient occasionally can remove the food particle with forced regurgitation. This extremely disagreeable and frightening form of dysphagia is a sword of Damocles hanging permanently over almost all patients who have EE. It substantially impairs the quality of life and may affect the patient's lifestyle, profession, and social contacts. The best way to prevent food impaction is to treat the underlying inflammation and to dilate relevant strictures. In contrast, there is no established medical treatment for the management of an acute blockade. Calcium-channel blockers, nitroglycerin, and spasmolytic analgesics have no proven value. If the blockade persists for more than 1 hour, the chance of self-resolution is small, and the patient should be referred to an emergency gastroenterology service. The impacted bolus must be removed with a flexible endoscope. (See the article by Aceves and colleagues, elsewhere in this issue.) Rigid esophagoscopy is strongly discouraged in patients who have EE because of the potential increased relevant risk of perforation, as discussed in the later section in this article on procedure-related complications and in the article by Aceves and colleagues, elsewhere in this issue.

Short-segment esophageal narrowing

Short-segment stenoses or so-called "esophageal strictures" are a further well-known and frequently observed complication of EE in both children[15] and in adults.[2,12,28,34] One radiographic study documented strictures in 10 of 13 patients who had EE (77%),[2] and another endoscopic analysis identified strictures in 17 of 31 (57%) adult patients who had EE.[12] Endoscopy generally is considered more sensitive than radiography in detecting short-segment narrowing.[27] Despite the assumption that stricture formation represents a long-term sequela of EE, an analysis of one pediatric series demonstrates that strictures can occur even early in the course of EE.[15] The risk of stricture formation may be much lower in children than in adults, because in a barium contrast study in a large series of 381 pediatric patients, Liacouras and colleagues[16] found esophageal narrowing in only 24 patients (~ 6%). EE-associated strictures may have the appearance of a solitary ring, of a short ringed segment, of a short homogenous narrowed segment, or of normal-appearing mucosa that resist endoscope passage (**Fig. 2**).[35]

An analysis of 10 patients who had steroid-refractory strictures revealed that narrowed segments appear solitary or multiple and may involve the proximal, the middle, and/or the distal esophagus without any predilection.[36] The degree of the stenosis may vary from a mild form, found incidentally, to severe stenosis evoking severe swallowing disturbances and impairing endoscope passage.

If strictures lead to symptoms, treatment is indicated. As a first step, the author and colleagues recommend that several biopsies be taken from the strictured segment to distinguish inflammatory from fibrotic strictures to exclude a malignant stenosis. If endoscopy and histology indicate an inflammatory stricture, the author and colleagues recommend a course of topical corticosteroids (eg, 2 mg oral fluticasone, daily, for at least 4 weeks) as a first-line therapy. To assess the efficacy of the treatment, a clinical and endoscopic/histologic follow-up examination is recommended.

For strictures refractory to this medication or for fibrotic strictures, gentle dilation is indicated. This procedure can be performed safely and usually leads to prompt symptom relief for up to 1 year. The underlying inflammation is not influenced by dilation, however. The role of anti-inflammatory drugs in primary and secondary prevention of stricture formation requires further clarification. (See the articles by Liacouras; Aceves and colleagues elsewhere in this issue.)

Long-segment esophageal narrowing

In EE, the narrowing also may encompass the full length of the esophagus. To date, this is the most severe disease-inherent complication of long-standing EE. Two different forms of long-segment stenoses have been reported. The literature refers to the first form as "trachealization",[37] "corrugated ringed esophagus",[38] "multiple-concentric ringed esophagus",[39] or "feline esophagus".[40] All these terms describe an esophagus that has multiple, concentric, trachea-like and sometimes subtle and inconstant rings. The second form is described as "small-caliber esophagus"[41] and "congenital too small esophagi".[42] These descriptions refer to a diffuse, non-ringed, long-segment esophageal stenosis. It has not yet clear why the narrowing process in EE may differ in size and type. This second form may be more apparent on an esophagram when the physiologic contractions that normally are visible are lost because of the severe underlying inflammation and remodeling. The therapeutic strategy for patients who have a long-segment stenosis is comparable to that discussed previously for short-segment stenoses. In accordance with the literature, the author and colleagues also recommend medical therapy first be undertaken for

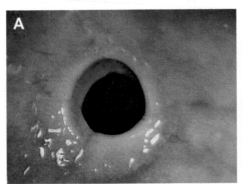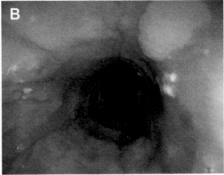

Fig. 2. Eosinophilic esophagitis with strictures of different sizes and types. (*A*) Endoscopic picture from a 27-year-old man who had EE and a 7-year history of dysphagia. The two neighboring rings in the proximal esophagus led to severe obstruction, impassable even with a small-caliber pediatric endoscope. (*B*) Endoscopic picture from a 54-year-old man who had EE and an 8-year history of dysphagia. The narrow mid-esophageal segment shows a cobblestone- and ring-like structure not passable with a standard endoscope before therapy.

long-segment stenoses and that dilation be considered only in patients who do not respond to anti-inflammatory treatment.[40] (See the article by Aceves and colleagues elsewhere in this issue.)

Eosinophilic esophagitis may lead to secondary gastroesophageal reflux disease

In addition to the leading symptom of dysphagia, up to 30% of patients who have EE experience retrosternal pain that is not associated with the act of swallowing.[27,43] Clinically, it may be difficult to distinguish between pain resulting from the eosinophilic inflammation and pain resulting from a co-existing reflux disease (eg, GERD). The definition of EE therefore includes the proviso that the symptoms must persist despite a prolonged therapy with proton-pump inhibitors.[4] In addition, reflux often is excluded by pH-monitoring studies before a diagnosis of EE finally is established.[44] It is common, however, to find that typical reflux symptoms that do respond to acid-suppressive medication appear during the long-term course of EE. In their case series, Remedios and colleagues[14] found that among 26 adult patients who had EE, 10 had coexisting reflux disease that had been confirmed by pH monitoring. Furthermore, based on motility studies, the authors found that 8 of the 10 patients who had coexisting reflux also had a dysfunction of the lower esophageal sphincter with reduced pressure. In contrast, endoscopically, no typical signs of a reflux disease, such as hiatal hernia, were reported. (See the article by Fox elsewhere in this issue.) In summary, clinical observations and the findings from the study by Remedios and colleagues[14] suggest that, in EE, the chronic inflammation can lead to a dysfunction of the lower esophageal sphincter and thus to a clinically relevant, secondary reflux disease.

Eosinophilic esophagitis may predispose a patient to esophageal infections

On endoscopic or histologic examination it common to encounter *Candida albicans* infection in patients who have EE. Fungal infections are a well-known complication of therapy with topical corticosteroids, but, as illustrated in **Fig. 3**, esophageal candidiasis also can occur spontaneously in patients who have EE.

In addition, EE also may lead to viral infections of the esophagus, as demonstrated in **Fig. 4**.

These two cases illustrate that, in pre-existing EE, fungal and viral infections may occur even in the absence of risk factors such as therapy with topical corticosteroids or immunosuppressive conditions.

Eosinophilic esophagitis may lead to spontaneous esophageal rupture (Boerhaave's syndrome)

To date, three cases have been reported in which patients who had EE experienced a spontaneously occurring transmural esophageal rupture.[45–47] Two patients experienced the rupture during an acute episode with nausea and repeated vomiting, probably caused by a gastrointestinal infection. In the third patient the rupture occurred during repeated retching caused by an impacted food bolus. All patients had suffered from pre-existing dysphagia for years, but the diagnosis of EE had not been made before the esophageal rupture occurred. These three cases broaden the clinical spectrum and extend the risk profile of EE.

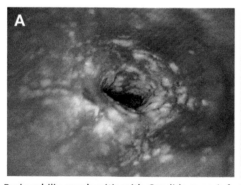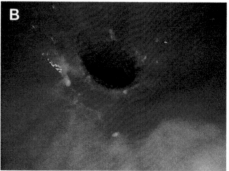

Fig. 3. Eosinophilic esophagitis with Candida superinfection. (*A*) Endoscopic picture of a 23-year-old man who had EE and a history of allergic rhinitis and dysphagia of 9 years' duration. The endoscopically noted inflamed mucosa from the distal third of the esophagus was covered by white membranes. Histology confirmed a *Candida albicans* infection that was treated with a topical antifungal medication and led to improvement of dysphagia. (*B*) Six weeks later, endoscopy revealed a mild stenosis with a few white exudates. Biopsies from this segment showed the typical sings of EE, with a peak infiltration of 38 eosinophils per HPF, thereby confirming the diagnosis of EE for which topical corticosteroids were administered.

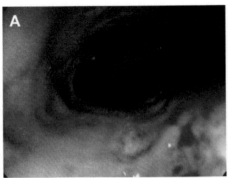
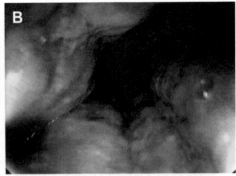

Fig. 4. Eosinophilic esophagitis with Herpes simplex superinfection. (*A*) Endoscopic pictures from a 25-year-old woman with a 9-year history of EE. After being almost completely symptom-free without any therapy for several years, the patient experienced acute severe odynophagia, fever, and malaise, almost preventing the ingestion even of liquids. An emergency upper endoscopy showed a homogenously severely inflamed esophageal mucosa with deep, ring-shaped ulcers. Histology revealed an acute, severe inflammation with a pure neutrophilic infiltration. Serologic analyses revealed a high antibody titer for Herpes simplex virus type 1 IgM. Herpes esophagitis was diagnosed, and antiviral medication commenced. Symptoms disappeared over the next few days. (*B*) Endoscopic control 5 weeks later showed an irregular surface of the esophageal mucosa but also the typical sings of EE in the form of extensive white exudates and some red furrows. Histologically, a dense eosinophilic infiltration of the esophageal epithelium with microabscesses was found.

Patients who have long-standing EE therefore are at risk for retching-induced esophageal rupture. Although their underlying diagnosis has not been identified, all three patients were treated surgically in accordance with established guidelines for esophageal perforations[48] and recovered well. EE-associated esophageal rupture therefore can be managed according to established standards and does not require a special procedure. Because Boerhaave's syndrome may be the first presentation of EE, the author and colleagues recommend that, after the patient has recovered from this life-threatening event, an upper endoscopy should be performed with biopsy sampling from the proximal and the distal esophagus to assess for mucosal inflammation that may benefit from medical or nutritional treatments.

Procedure-Related Complications

Procedure-related complications also are discussed in the article by Aceves and colleagues, elsewhere in this issue.

Peri- and postprocedural pain

It is frequently observed that, in contrast to other patients, patients who have EE experience retrosternal pain during or even after a completely uneventful endoscopy[35] or during biopsy sampling. Furthermore, it is well known that after dilation of EE-related esophageal stenoses, patients may suffer from severe retrosternal pain, mostly associated with swallowing, for several days. This experience contrasts with the retrosternal pain unassociated with swallowing, which is a prevalent EE symptom.

An analysis of efficacy and risks associated with the dilation of corticosteroid-refractory EE stenosis found that 6 of 10 patients suffered from severe odynophagia for an average of 2 days (range, 1–3 days).[36] Peri- and postprocedural retrosternal pain therefore is a common and almost EE-specific problem.

This abnormal behavior of the EE esophagi must be taken into account if invasive examinations (eg, endoscopies, endoscopic ultrasound examinations, and manometric studies) and endoscopic therapies are planned. This behavior has the following practical consequences:

1. All procedures must be performed extremely gently.
2. Procedures should be performed under sedation.
3. The patient must be informed about this potential complication before the procedure is performed.

Procedure-related esophageal perforation

The esophagus is a hidden organ, and invasive procedures, such as upper endoscopy, frequently are required for diagnostic or surveillance purposes that are usually accompanied by a small risk of perforation. In contrast, patients who have EE often require therapeutic procedures, including removal of impacted food or dilation of strictures, and have a substantially increased risk of mucosal renting or even perforation.[40] This particularity is caused by a remodeling process[30] that results in an extremely fragile, inelastic, and rigid esophageal

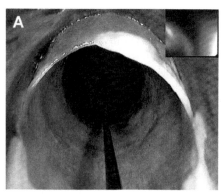 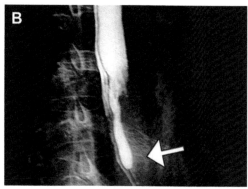

Fig. 5. Eosinophilic esophagitis with esophageal dissection. (*A*) Flexible endoscopy in a 37-year-old woman who had a 20-year history of dysphagia, performed immediately after an ear, nose, and throat surgeon's attempt to remove an impacted bolus using rigid esophagoscopy. A complete and circular dissection of the esophageal wall can be seen. (*B*) Esophagography of the same patient showing a huge dissection channel (*white arrow*) with a compression of the remaining esophageal lumen.

wall structure that tears easily.[49] To date, four esophageal perforations have been reported. One occurred after simple passage of the endoscope,[40] one occurred after dilation,[50] and two developed during an attempt to remove impacted food by rigid endoscopy.[47] All patients had intense chest pain immediately after the procedure, and the clinically suspected perforation was confirmed by CT scan, which revealed either a frank perforation with pneumomediastinum and pneumoperitoneum or a sealed perforation with intramural air in the esophagus. All four patients were treated conservatively and recovered completely without any further complications. **Fig. 5** illustrates this life-threatening complication in a patient in whom a procedure-related perforation occurred during an ear, nose, and throat surgeon's attempt to remove impacted food with rigid esophagoscopy.

In summary, at least four procedure-related esophageal perforations have been reported. Half of these life-threatening complications occurred during a rigid esophagoscopy for removing impacted food. Intense retrosternal and upper abdominal pain after a diagnostic or therapeutic procedure is performed should raise the suspicion of perforation. All four cases were manageable without surgery. Close monitoring under ICU conditions, nasogastric intubation, total parenteral nutrition, and parenteral application of antibiotics may be necessary. Of note, rigid esophagoscopy seems to be impose increased risks of perforation than flexible endoscopy and should be strongly discouraged in patients who have EE.

SUMMARY

Based on the information available, it is clear that EE is a chronic and persisting or a chronic and relapsing disease that, left untreated, probably leads to irreversible structural alterations of the esophagus. Nevertheless, the knowledge of the natural history of EE and of the underlying mechanisms leading to the perpetuation of this inflammation[11] is still limited, and many aspects and complications may still be unknown. To learn more about the course and the complications of this recently described disorder, vigorous efforts are needed to carry out properly designed, long-term natural history studies in pediatric and adult patients.

ACKNOWLEDGMENTS

The author and his colleagues would like to thank their Swiss gastroenterology colleagues for referring patients to our EE clinic in Olten. The author also thanks Stephan Bucher for his critical review and comments regarding the section on study design, Kathleen Bucher for her competent editorial work, and Christian Bussmann and Hanspeter Spichtin for their excellent pathology contribution.

REFERENCES

1. Attwood SE, Smyrk TC, Demeester TR, et al. Esophageal eosinophilia with dysphagia. A distinct clinicopathologic syndrome. Dig Dis Sci 1993;38:109–16.
2. Vitellas KM, Bennett WF, Bova JG, et al. Idiopathic eosinophilic esophagitis. Radiology 1993;186:789–93.
3. Straumann A, Spichtin HP, Bernoulli R, et al. Idiopathic eosinophilic esophagitis: a frequently overlooked disease with typical clinical aspects and discrete endoscopic findings [in German with English abstract]. Schweiz Med Wochenschr 1994; 124:1419–29.

4. Furuta GT, Straumann A. The pathogenesis and management of eosinophilic oesophagitis. Aliment Pharmacol Ther 2006;24:173–82.

5. Desai TK, Stecevic V, Chang CH, et al. Association of eosinophilic inflammation with esophageal food impaction in adults. Gastrointest Endosc 2005;61: 795–801.

6. Noel RJ, Putnam PE, Rothenberg ME. Eosinophilic esophagitis. N Engl J Med 2004;351:940–1.

7. Kim DJ, Lifschitz CH, Bonis PA. Eosinophilic esophagitis. In: UpToDate in gastroenterology and hepatology. 2006;vol. 10/06.

8. Hulley SB, Cummings SR, Browner WS, et al. Designing clinical research. 3rd edition. Philadelphia Baltimore, New York, London, Buenos Aires, Hong Kong, Sidney, Tokyo: Lippincott Wiliams & Wilkins, Wolters Kluwer; 2007. p. 97–106.

9. Straumann A, Spichtin HP, Grize L, et al. Natural history of primary eosinophilic esophagitis: a follow-up of 30 adult patients for up to 11.5 years. Gastroenterology 2003;125:1660–9.

10. Konikoff MR, Noel RJ, Blanchard C. A randomized, double-blind, placebo-controlled trial of fluticasone propionate for pediatric eosinophilic esophagitis. Gastroenterology 2006;131:1381–91.

11. Furuta GT, Liacouras CA, Collins MH, et al. Eosinophilic esophagitis in children and adults: a systematic review and consensus recommendations for diagnosis and treatment. Gastroenterology 2007; 133:1342–63.

12. Croese J, Fairley SK, Masson JW, et al. Clinical and endoscopic features of eosinophilic esophagitis in adults. Gastrointest Endosc 2003;58:516–22.

13. Straumann A, Spichtin HP, Bucher KA, et al. Eosinophilic esophagitis: red on microscopy, white on endoscopy. Digestion 2004;70:109–16.

14. Remedios M, Campbell C, Jones DM, et al. Eosinophilic esophagitis in adults: clinical, endoscopic, histologic findings, and response to treatment with fluticasone propionate. Gastrointest Endosc 2006; 63:3–12.

15. Khan S, Orenstein SR, Di Lorenzo C, et al. Eosinophilic esophagitis: strictures, impactions, dysphagia. Dig Dis Sci 2003;48:22–9.

16. Liacouras CA, Spergel JM, Ruchelli E, et al. Eosinophilic esophagitis: a 10-year experience in 381 children. Clin Gastroenterol Hepatol 2005;3:1198–206.

17. Rothenberg ME. Eosinophilic gastrointestinal disorders (EGID). J Allergy Clin Immunol 2004;113:11–28.

18. Fogg MI, Ruchelli E, Spergel JM. Pollen and eosinophilic esophagitis [letter]. J Allergy Clin Immunol 2003;112:796–7.

19. Wang FY, Gupta SK, Fitzgerald JF. Is there a seasonal variation in the incidence or intensity of allergic eosinophilic esophagitis in newly diagnosed children? J Clin Gastroenterol 2007;41:451–3.

20. Walsh SV, Antonioli DA, Goldman H, et al. Allergic esophagitis in children: a clinicopathological entity. Am J Surg Pathol 1999;23:390–6.

21. Dobbins JW, Sheahan DG. Behar J.Eosinophilic gastroenteritis with esophageal involvement. Gastroenterology 1977;72:1312–6.

22. Mahajan L, Wyllie R, Petras R, et al. Idiopathic eosinophilic esophagitis with stricture formation in a patient with long-standing eosinophilic gastroenteritis. Gastrointest Endosc 1997;46:557–60.

23. Schmid-Grendelmeier P, Altznauer F, Fischer B, et al. Eosinophils express functional IL-13 in eosinophilic inflammatory diseases. J Immunol 2002;169:1021–7.

24. Reed CE. The natural history of asthma in adults: the problem of irreversibility. J Allergy Clin Immunol 1999;103:539–47.

25. Cho JY, Miller M, Baik KJ, et al. Immunostimulatory DNA inhibits transforming growth factor-beta expression and airway remodeling. Am J Respir Cell Mol Biol 2004;30:651–61.

26. Mishra A, Hogan SP, Brandt EB, et al. An etiological role for aeroallergens and eosinophils in experimental esophagitis. J Clin Invest 2001;107:83–90.

27. Potter JW, Saeian K, Staff D, et al. Eosinophilic esophagitis in adults: an emerging problem with unique esophageal features. Gastrointest Endosc 2004;59:355–61.

28. Parfitt JR, Gregor JC, Suskin NG, et al. Eosinophilic esophagitis in adults: distinguishing features from gastroesophageal reflux disease: a study of 41 patients. Mod Pathol 2006;19:90–6.

29. Mueller S, Aigner T, Neureiter D, et al. Eosinophil infiltration and degranulation in oesophageal mucosa from adult patients with eosinophilic oesophagitis: a retrospective and comparative study on pathological biopsy. J Clin Pathol 2006;59:1175–80.

30. Aceves SS, Newbury RO, Dohil R, et al. Esophageal remodeling in pediatric eosinophilic esophagitis. J Allergy Clin Immunol 2007;119:206–12.

31. Fox VL, Nurko S, Teitelbaum, et al. High-resolution EUS in children with eosinophilic "allergic" esophagitis. Gastrointest Endosc 2003;57:30–6.

32. Bauer S, Schaub N, Dommann-Scherrer CC, et al. Long-term outcome of idiopathic hypereosinophilic syndrome — transition to eosinophilic gastroenteritis and clonal expansion of T-cells. Eur J Gastroenterol Hepatol 1996;8:181–5.

33. Simon HU, Plötz SG, Dummer R, et al. Abnormal clones of T cells producing interleukin-5 in idiopathic eosinophilia. N Engl J Med 1999;341:1112–20.

34. Feczko PJ, Halpert RD, Zonca M. Radiographic abnormalities in eosinophilic esophagitis. Gastrointest Radiol 1985;10:321–4.

35. Van Rosendaal GM, Anderson MA, Diamant NE. Eosinophilic esophagitis: case report and clinical perspective. Am J Gastroenterol 1997;92:1054–6.

36. Schoepfer AM, Gschossmann J, Scheurer U, et al. Esophageal strictures in eosinophilic esophagitis: dilation is an effective and safe therapeutic alternative after failure of topical corticosteroids. Endoscopy 2007, in press.

37. Langdon DE. "Congenital" esophageal stenosis, corrugated ringed esophagus, and eosinophilic esophagitis. Am J Gastroenterol 2000;95:2123–4.

38. Langdon DE. Corrugated ringed esophagus. Am J Gastroenterol 1993;88:1461.

39. Siafakas CG, Ryan CK, Brown MR, et al. Multiple esophageal rings: an association with eosinophilic esophagitis: case report and review of the literature. Am J Gastroenterol 2000;95:1572–5.

40. Kaplan M, Mutlu EA, Jakate S, et al. Endoscopy in eosinophilic esophagitis: "feline" esophagus and perforation risk. Clin Gastroenterol Hepatol 2003;1: 433–7.

41. Vasilopoulos S, Murphy P, Auerbach A, et al. The small-caliber esophagus: an unappreciated cause of dysphagia for solids in patients with eosinophilic esophagitis. Gastrointest Endosc 2002;55: 99–106.

42. Langdon DE. Corrugated ringed and too small esophagi. Am J Gastroenterol 1999;94:542–3.

43. Orenstein SR, Shalaby TM, DiLorenzo C, et al. The spectrum of pediatric eosinophilic esophagitis beyond infancy: a clinical series of 30 children. Am J Gastroenterol 2000;95:1422–30.

44. Kelly KJ, Lazenby AJ, Rowe PC, et al. Eosinophilic esophagitis attributed to gastroesophageal reflux: improvement with an amino acid-based formula. Gastroenterology 1995;109:1503–12.

45. Riou PJ, Nicholson AG, Pastorino U. Esophageal rupture in a patient with idiopathic eosinophilic esophagitis. Ann Thorac Surg 1996;62:1854–6.

46. Cohen MS, Kaufmann AB, Palazzo JP, et al. An audit of endoscopic complications in adult eosinophilic esophagitis. Clin Gastroenterol Hepatol 2007;5:1149–53.

47. Straumann A, Bussmann C, Zuber M, et al. Eosinophilic Esophagitis: Analysis of food impaction and perforation in 251 adult patients. Clin Gastroenterol Hepatol 2007 [under review].

48. Tilanus HW, Bossuyt P, Schattenkerk ME, et al. Treatment of oesophageal perforation: a multivariate analysis. Br J Surg 1991;78:582–5.

49. Straumann A, Rossi L, Simon HU, et al. Fragility of the esophageal mucosa: a pathognomonic endoscopic sign of primary eosinophilic eesophagitis? Gastrointest Endosc 2003;57:407–12.

50. Eisenbach C, Merle U, Schirmacher P. Perforation of the esophagus after dilation treatment of dysphagia in a patient with eosinophilic esophagitis. Endoscopy 2006;38:E43–4.

Index

Thorac Surg Clin 21 (2011) 589–595
doi:10.1016/S1547-4127(11)00122-8

thoracic.theclinics.com

United States Postal Service

Statement of Ownership, Management, and Circulation
(All Periodicals Publications Except Requester Publications)

1. Publication Title	2. Publication Number	3. Filing Date
Thoracic Surgery Clinics	0 1 3 - 1 2 6	9/16/11

4. Issue Frequency	5. Number of Issues Published Annually	6. Annual Subscription Price
Feb, May, Aug, Nov	4	$295.00

7. Complete Mailing Address of Known Office of Publication (Not printer) (Street, city, county, state, and ZIP+4®)

Elsevier Inc.
360 Park Avenue South
New York, NY 10010-1710

Contact Person
Stephen Bushing

Telephone (Include area code)
215-239-3688

8. Complete Mailing Address of Headquarters or General Business Office of Publisher (Not printer)

Elsevier Inc., 360 Park Avenue South, New York, NY 10010-1710

9. Full Names and Complete Mailing Addresses of Publisher, Editor, and Managing Editor (Do not leave blank)
Publisher (Name and complete mailing address)

Kim Murphy, Elsevier, Inc., 1600 John F. Kennedy Blvd. Suite 1800, Philadelphia, PA 19103-2899

Editor (Name and complete mailing address)

Barbara Cohen-Kligerman, Elsevier, Inc., 1600 John F. Kennedy Blvd. Suite 1800, Philadelphia, PA 19103-2899

Managing Editor (Name and complete mailing address)

Barbara Cohen-Kligerman, Elsevier, Inc., 1600 John F. Kennedy Blvd. Suite 1800, Philadelphia, PA 19103-2899

10. Owner (Do not leave blank. If the publication is owned by a corporation, give the name and address of the corporation immediately followed by the names and addresses of all stockholders owning or holding 1 percent or more of the total amount of stock. If not owned by a corporation, give the names and addresses of the individual owners. If owned by a partnership or other unincorporated firm, give its name and address as well as those of each individual owner. If the publication is published by a nonprofit organization, give its name and address.)

Full Name	Complete Mailing Address
Wholly owned subsidiary of	4520 East-West Highway
Reed/Elsevier, US holdings	Bethesda, MD 20814

11. Known Bondholders, Mortgagees, and Other Security Holders Owning or Holding 1 Percent or More of Total Amount of Bonds, Mortgages, or Other Securities. If none, check box ☐ None

Full Name	Complete Mailing Address
N/A	

12. Tax Status (For completion by nonprofit organizations authorized to mail at nonprofit rates) (Check one)
The purpose, function, and nonprofit status of this organization and the exempt status for federal income tax purposes:
☐ Has Not Changed During Preceding 12 Months
☐ Has Changed During Preceding 12 Months (Publisher must submit explanation of change with this statement)

PS Form 3526, September 2007 (Page 1 of 3 (Instructions Page 3)) PSN 7530-01-000-9931 PRIVACY NOTICE: See our Privacy policy in www.usps.com

13. Publication Title		14. Issue Date for Circulation Data Below
Thoracic Surgery Clinics		August 2011

15. Extent and Nature of Circulation			Average No. Copies Each Issue During Preceding 12 Months	No. Copies of Single Issue Published Nearest to Filing Date
a. Total Number of Copies (Net press run)			1243	1063
b. Paid Circulation (By Mail and Outside the Mail)	(1)	Mailed Outside-County Paid Subscriptions Stated on PS Form 3541. (Include paid distribution above nominal rate, advertiser's proof copies, and exchange copies)	560	522
	(2)	Mailed In-County Paid Subscriptions Stated on PS Form 3541 (Include paid distribution above nominal rate, advertiser's proof copies, and exchange copies)		
	(3)	Paid Distribution Outside the Mails Including Sales Through Dealers and Carriers, Street Vendors, Counter Sales, and Other Paid Distribution Outside USPS®	206	210
	(4)	Paid Distribution by Other Classes Mailed Through the USPS (e.g. First-Class Mail®)		
c. Total Paid Distribution (Sum of 15b (1), (2), (3), and (4))		►	766	732
d. Free or Nominal Rate Distribution (By Mail and Outside the Mail)	(1)	Free or Nominal Rate Outside-County Copies Included on PS Form 3541	49	56
	(2)	Free or Nominal Rate In-County Copies Included on PS Form 3541		
	(3)	Free or Nominal Rate Copies Mailed at Other Classes Through the USPS (e.g. First-Class Mail)		
	(4)	Free or Nominal Rate Distribution Outside the Mail (Carriers or other means)		
e. Total Free or Nominal Rate Distribution (Sum of 15d (1), (2), (3) and (4))		►	49	56
f. Total Distribution (Sum of 15c and 15e)		►	815	788
g. Copies not Distributed (See instructions to publishers #4 (page #3))		►	428	275
h. Total (Sum of 15f and g)		►	1243	1063
i. Percent Paid (15c divided by 15f times 100)		►	93.99%	92.89%

16. Publication of Statement of Ownership
If the publication is a general publication, publication of this statement is required. Will be printed
in the November 2011 issue of this publication.   ☐ Publication not required

17. Signature and Title of Editor, Publisher, Business Manager, or Owner

Stephen R. Bushing – Inventory/Distribution Coordinator   Date: September 16, 2011

I certify that all information furnished on this form is true and complete. I understand that anyone who furnishes false or misleading information on this form or who omits material or information requested on the form may be subject to criminal sanctions (including fines and imprisonment) and/or civil sanctions (including civil penalties).

PS Form 3526, September 2007 (Page 2 of 3)

Moving?

Make sure your subscription moves with you!

To notify us of your new address, find your **Clinics Account Number** (located on your mailing label above your name), and contact customer service at:

Email: journalscustomerservice-usa@elsevier.com

800-654-2452 (subscribers in the U.S. & Canada)
314-447-8871 (subscribers outside of the U.S. & Canada)

Fax number: 314-447-8029

Elsevier Health Sciences Division
Subscription Customer Service
3251 Riverport Lane
Maryland Heights, MO 63043

*To ensure uninterrupted delivery of your subscription, please notify us at least 4 weeks in advance of move.

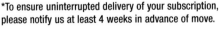

Printed and bound by CPI Group (UK) Ltd, Croydon, CR0 4YY

03/10/2024

01040351-0010